The Best Mediterranean Recipes

A Complete Collection of Recipes to Start Your
Mediterranean Diet and Manage Your Weight

America Best Recipes

Table of contents

Mediterranean Baked Chickpeas

Preparation Time: 15 minutes

Cooking Time: 15 minute

Servings: 6

Ingredients :

- 1 tbsp. extra-virgin olive oil
- ½ medium onion, chopped
- 3 garlic cloves, chopped
- 2 tsp. smoked paprika
- ¼ tsp. ground cumin
- 4 cups halved cherry tomatoes
- 2 (15-oz.) cans chickpeas, drained and rinsed
- ½ cup plain, unsweetened, full-fat Greek yogurt, for serving
- 1 cup crumbled feta, for serving

Directions:

2. Preheat the oven to 425°F.

3. In an oven-safe sauté pan or skillet, heat the oil over medium heat and sauté the onion and garlic. Cook for about 5 minutes, until softened and fragrant. Stir in the paprika and cumin and cook for 2 minutes. Stir in the tomatoes and chickpeas.

4. Bring to a simmer for 5 to 10 minutes before placing in the oven.

5. Roast in oven for 25 to 30 minutes, until bubbling and thickened. To serve, top with Greek yogurt and feta.

Nutrition:

Calories: 330;

Carbs: 75.4g;

Protein: 9.0g;

Fat: 18.5g

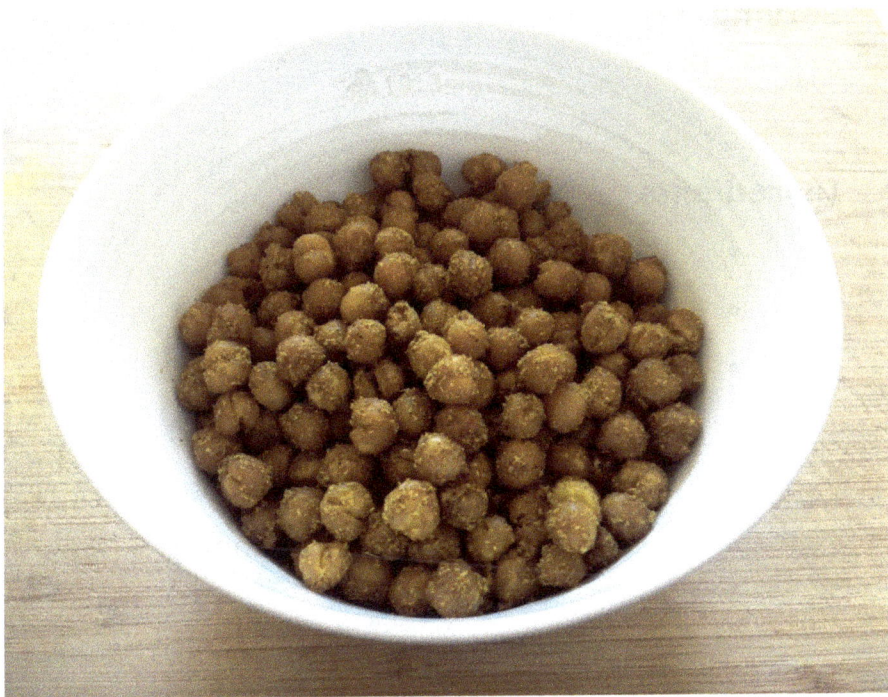

Falafel Bites

Preparation Time: 10 minutes

Cooking Time: 15 minute

Servings: 4

Ingredients :

- 1 2/3 cups falafel mix
- 1¼ cups water
- Extra-virgin olive oil spray
- 1 tbsp. Pickled Onions (optional)
- 1 tbsp. Pickled Turnips (optional)
- 2 tbsp. Tzatziki Sauce (optional)

Directions:

1. In a large bowl, carefully stir the falafel mix into the water. Mix well. Let stand 15 minutes to absorb the water. Form mix into 1-inch balls and arrange on a baking sheet.
2. Preheat the broiler to high.

3. Take the balls and flatten slightly with your thumb (so they won't roll around on the baking sheet). Spray with olive oil, and then broil for 2 to 3 minutes on each side, until crispy and brown.

4. To fry the falafel, fill a pot with ½ inch of cooking oil and heat over medium-high heat to 375°F. Fry the balls for about 3 minutes, until brown and crisp. Drain on paper towels and serve with pickled onions, pickled turnips, and tzatziki sauce (if using).

Nutrition:

Calories: 530;

Carbs: 95.4g;

Protein: 8.0g;

Fat: 18.5g

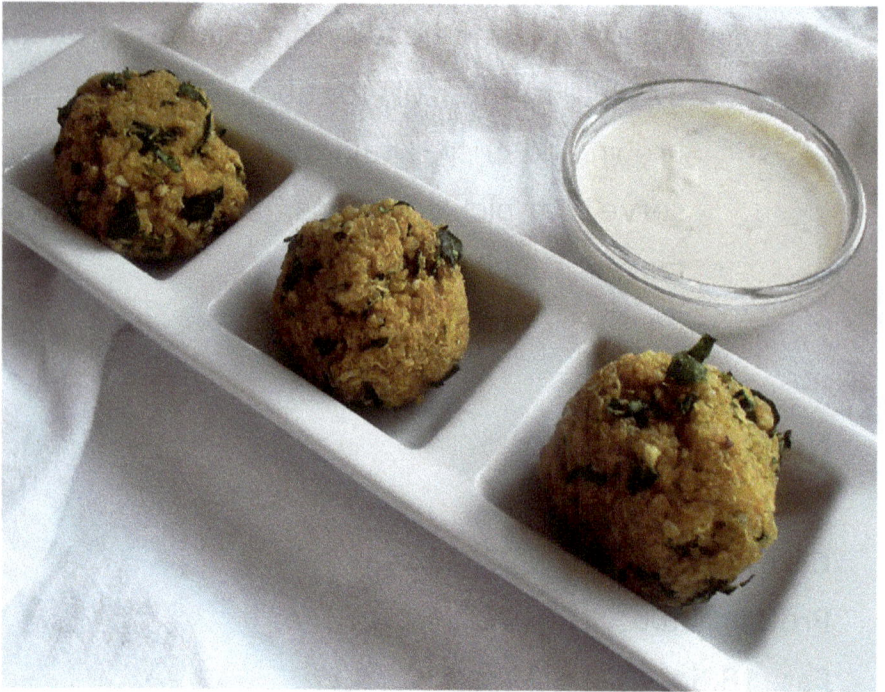

Quick Vegetable Kebabs

Preparation Time: 15 minutes

Cooking Time: 20 minute

Servings: 6

Ingredients :

- 4 medium red onions, peeled and sliced into 6 wedges
- 4 medium zucchini, cut into 1-inch-thick slices
- 4 bell peppers, cut into 2-inch squares
- 2 yellow bell peppers, cut into 2-inch squares
- 2 orange bell peppers, cut into 2-inch squares
- 2 beefsteak tomatoes, cut into quarters
- 3 tbsp. Herbed Oil

Directions:

1. Preheat the oven or grill to medium-high or 350°F.
2. Thread 1 piece red onion, zucchini, different colored bell peppers, and tomatoes onto a skewer. Repeat until the skewer is full of vegetables, up to 2 inches away from the skewer end, and continue until all skewers are complete.
3. Put the skewers on a baking sheet and cook in the oven for 10 minutes or grill for 5 minutes on each side. The vegetables will be done with they reach your desired crunch or softness.
4. Remove the skewers from heat and drizzle with Herbed Oil.

Nutrition:

Calories: 235;

Carbs: 30.4g;

Protein: 8.0g;

Fat: 14.5g

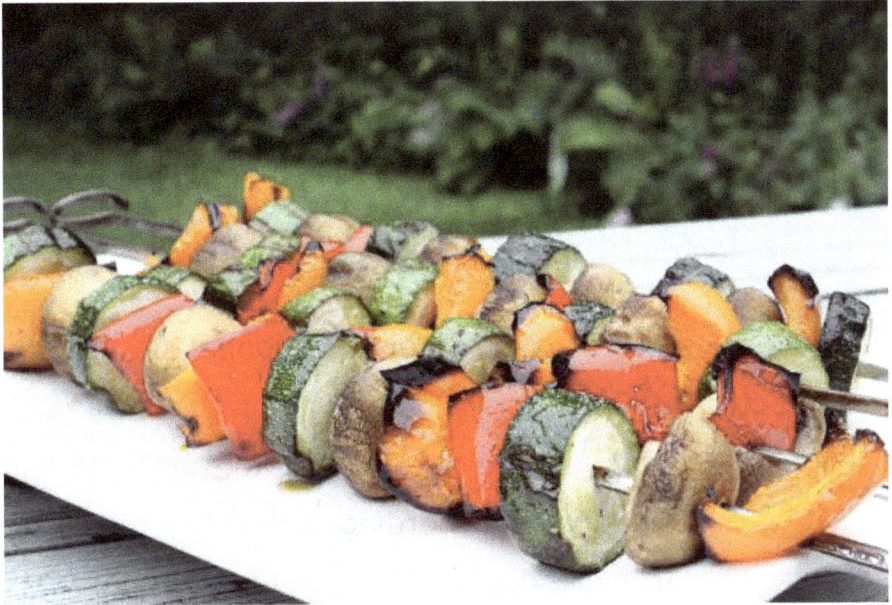

Tortellini in Red Pepper Sauce
Preparation Time: 15 minutes

Cooking Time: 10 minute

Servings: 4

Ingredients :

- 1 (16-oz.) container fresh cheese tortellini (usually green and white pasta)
- 1 (16-oz.) jar roasted red peppers, drained
- 1 tsp. garlic powder
- ¼ cup tahini
- 1 tbsp. red pepper oil (optional)

Directions:

1. Bring a large pot of water to a boil and cook the tortellini according to package directions.
2. In a blender, combine the red peppers with the garlic powder and process until smooth. Once blended, add the tahini until the sauce is thickened. If the sauce gets too thick, add up to 1 tbsp. red pepper oil (if using).
3. Once tortellini are cooked, drain and leave pasta in colander. Add the sauce to the bottom of the empty pot and heat for 2 minutes. Then, add the tortellini back into the

pot and cook for 2 more minutes. Serve and enjoy!

Nutrition:

Calories: 530;

Carbs: 95.4g;

Protein: 8.0g;

Fat: 18.5g

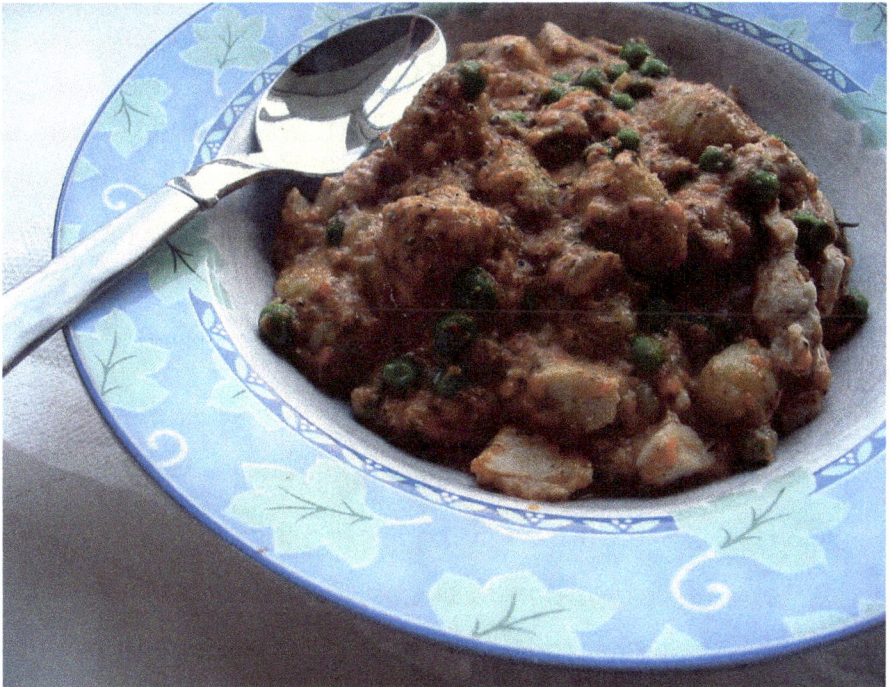

Freekeh, Chickpea, and Herb Salad

Preparation Time: 15 minutes

Cooking Time: 10 minute

Servings: 6

Ingredients :

- 1 (15-oz.) can chickpeas, rinsed and drained
- 1 cup cooked freekeh
- 1 cup thinly sliced celery
- 1 bunch scallions, both white and green parts, finely chopped
- ½ cup chopped fresh flat-leaf parsley
- ¼ cup chopped fresh mint
- 3 tbsp. chopped celery leaves
- ½ tsp. kosher salt
- 1/3 cup extra-virgin olive oil
- ¼ cup freshly squeezed lemon juice
- ¼ tsp. cumin seeds
- 1 tsp. garlic powder

Directions:

1. In a large bowl, combine the chickpeas, freekeh, celery, scallions, parsley, mint, celery leaves, and salt and toss lightly.

2. In a small bowl, whisk together the olive oil, lemon juice, cumin seeds, and garlic powder. Once combined, add to freekeh salad.

Nutrition:

Calories: 230;

Carbs: 25.4g;

Protein: 8.0g;

Fat: 18.5g

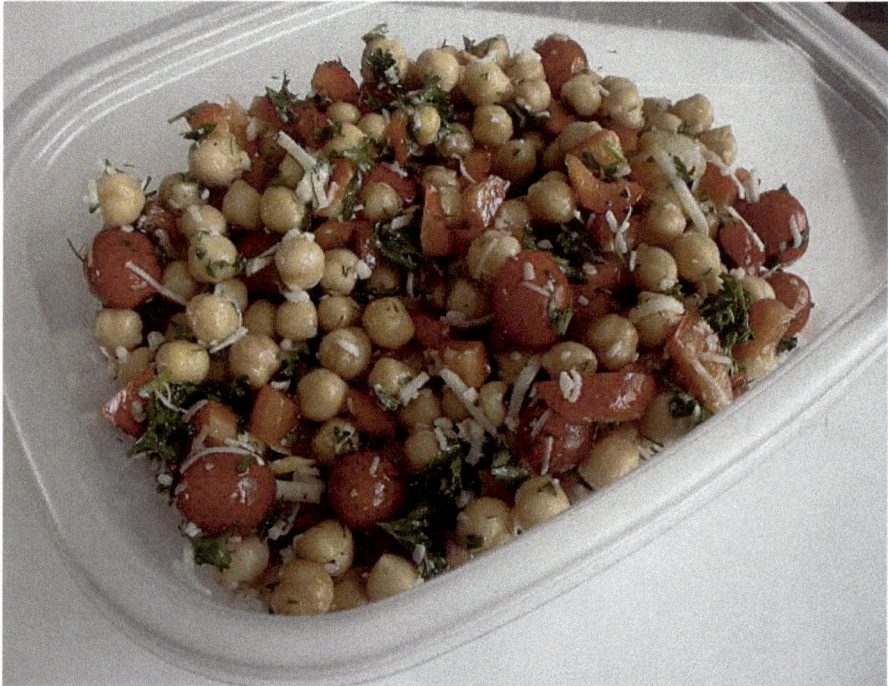

Kate's Warm Mediterranean Farro Bowl

Preparation Time: 15 minutes

Cooking Time: 10 minute

Servings: 4

Ingredients :

- 1/3 cup extra-virgin olive oil
- ½ cup chopped red bell pepper
- 1/3 cup chopped red onions
- 2 garlic cloves, minced
- 1 cup zucchini, cut in ½-inch slices
- ½ cup canned chickpeas, drained and rinsed
- ½ cup coarsely chopped artichokes
- 3 cups cooked farro
- Salt
- Freshly ground black pepper
- ¼ cup sliced olives, for serving (optional)
- ½ cup crumbled feta cheese, for serving (optional)
- 2 tbsp. fresh basil, chiffonade, for serving (optional)
- 3 tbsp. balsamic reduction, for serving (optional)

Directions:

1. In a large sauté pan or skillet, heat the oil over medium heat and sauté the pepper, onions, and garlic for about 5 minutes, until tender.
2. Add the zucchini, chickpeas, and artichokes, then stir and continue to sauté vegetables, approximately 5 more minutes, until just soft.
3. Stir in the cooked farro, tossing to combine and cooking enough to heat through. Season with salt and pepper and remove from the heat.
4. Transfer the contents of the pan into the serving vessels or bowls.
5. Top with olives, feta, and basil (if using). Drizzle with balsamic reduction (if using) to finish.

Nutrition:

Calories: 530;

Carbs: 95.4g;

Protein: 8.0g;

Fat: 13.5g

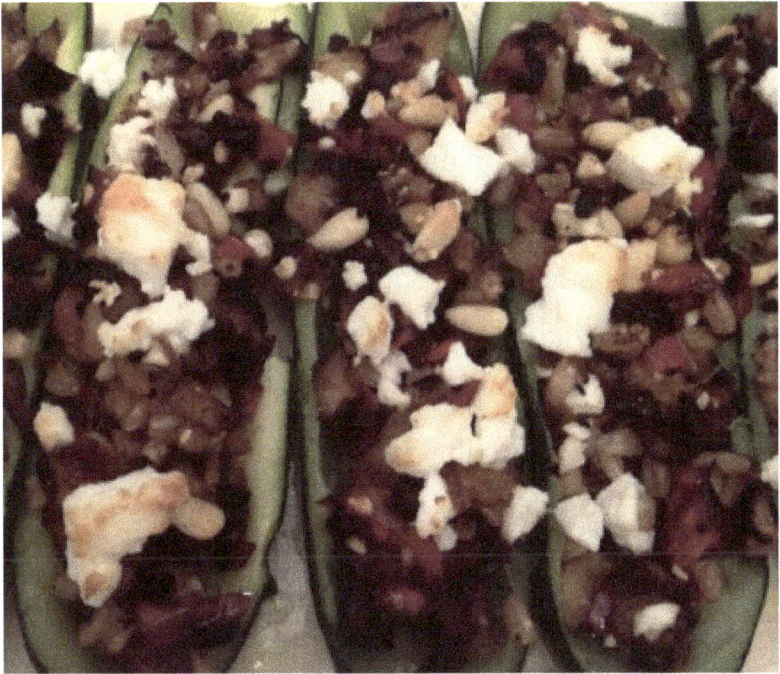

Creamy Chickpea Sauce with Whole-Wheat Fusilli

Preparation Time: 15 minutes

Cooking Time: 20 minute

Servings: 4

Ingredients :

- ¼ cup extra-virgin olive oil
- ½ large shallot, chopped
- 5 garlic cloves, thinly sliced
- 1 (15-oz.) can chickpeas, drained and rinsed, reserving ½ cup canning liquid
- Pinch red pepper flakes
- 1 cup whole-grain fusilli pasta
- ¼ tsp. salt
- 1/8 tsp. freshly ground black pepper
- ¼ cup shaved fresh Parmesan cheese
- ¼ cup chopped fresh basil
- 2 tsp. dried parsley
- 1 tsp. dried oregano
- Red pepper flakes

Directions:

1. In a medium pan, heat the oil over medium heat, and sauté the shallot and garlic for 3 to 5 minutes, until the garlic is golden. Add ¾ of

the chickpeas plus 2 tbsp. of liquid from the can, and bring to a simmer.

2. Remove from the heat, transfer into a standard blender, and blend until smooth. At this point, add the remaining chickpeas. Add more reserved chickpea liquid if it becomes thick.

3. Bring a large pot of salted water to a boil and cook pasta until al dente, about 8 minutes. Reserve ½ cup of the pasta water, drain the pasta, and return it to the pot.

4. Add the chickpea sauce to the hot pasta and add up to ¼ cup of the pasta water. You may need to add more pasta water to reach your desired consistency.

5. Place the pasta pot over medium heat and mix occasionally until the sauce thickens. Season with salt and pepper.

6. Serve, garnished with Parmesan, basil, parsley, oregano, and red pepper flakes.

Nutrition:

Calories: 230;

Carbs: 20.4g;

Protein: 8.0g;

Fat: 18.5g

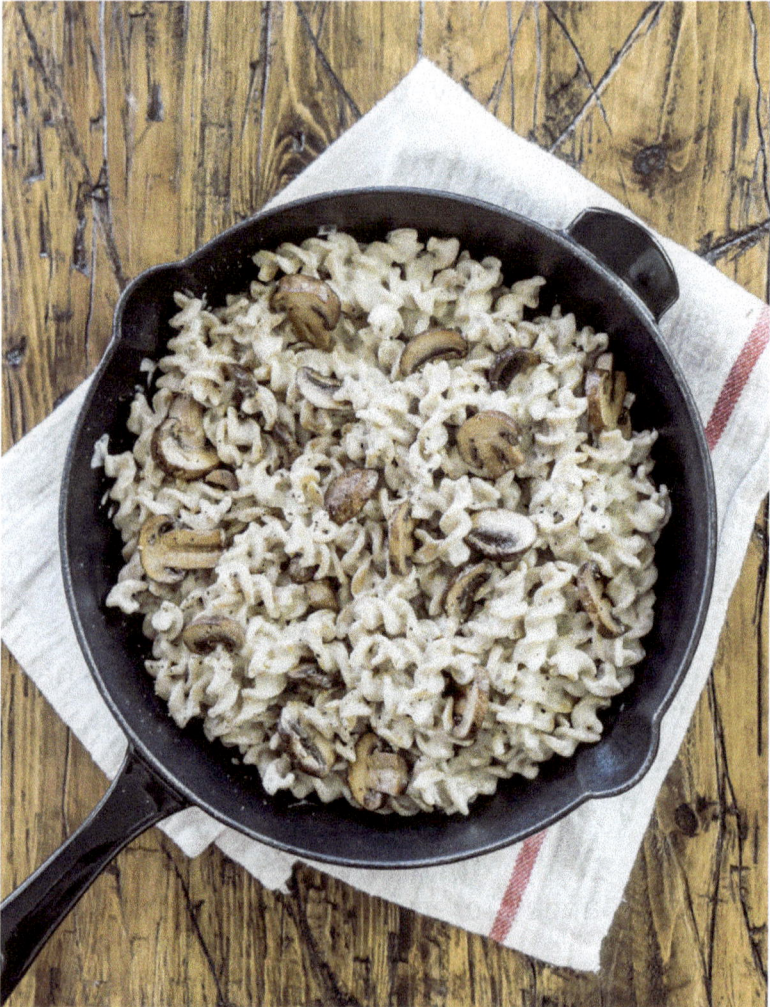

Linguine and Brussels sprouts

Preparation Time: 10 minutes

Cooking Time: 25 minute

Servings: 4

Ingredients :

- 8 oz. whole-wheat linguine
- 1/3 cup, plus 2 tbsp. extra-virgin olive oil, divided
- 1 medium sweet onion, diced
- 2 to 3 garlic cloves, smashed
- 8 oz. Brussels sprouts, chopped
- ½ cup chicken stock, as needed
- 1/3 cup dry white wine
- ½ cup shredded Parmesan cheese
- 1 lemon, cut in quarters

Directions:

1. Bring a large pot of water to a boil and cook the pasta according to package directions. Drain, reserving 1 cup of the pasta water. Mix the cooked pasta with 2 tbsp. of olive oil, then set aside.

2. In a large sauté pan or skillet, heat the remaining 1/3 cup of olive oil on medium heat. Add the onion to the pan and cook for about 5

minutes, until softened. Add the smashed garlic cloves and cook for 1 minute, until fragrant.

3.   Add the Brussels sprouts and cook covered for 15 minutes. Add chicken stock as needed to prevent burning. Once Brussels sprouts have wilted and are fork-tender, add white wine and cook down for about 7 minutes, until reduced.

4.   Add the pasta to the skillet and add the pasta water as needed.

5.   Serve with the Parmesan cheese and lemon for squeezing over the dish right before eating.

Nutrition:

Calories: 530;

Carbs: 95.4g;

Protein: 5.0g;

Fat: 16.5g

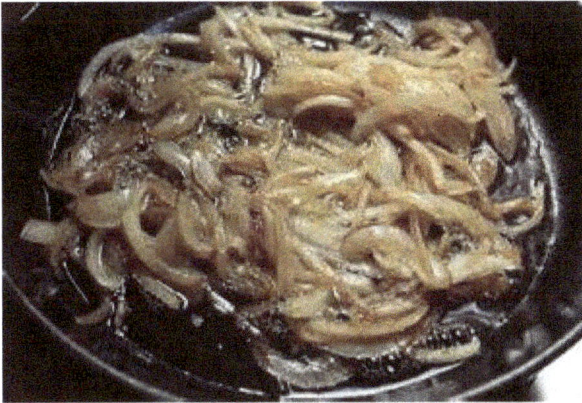

Peppers and Lentils Salad

Preparation Time: 10 minutes

Cooking Time: 0 minutes

Servings: 4

Ingredients:

- 14 oz. canned lentils, drained and rinsed
- 2 spring onions, chopped
- 1 red bell pepper, chopped
- 1 green bell pepper, chopped
- 1 tbsp. fresh lime juice
- 1/3 cup coriander, chopped
- 2 tsp. balsamic vinegar

Directions:

1. In a salad bowl, combine the lentils with the onions, bell peppers and the rest of the ingredients, toss and serve.

Nutrition: Calories 200, Fat 2.45g, Fiber 6.7g, Carbs 10.5g, Protein 5.6g

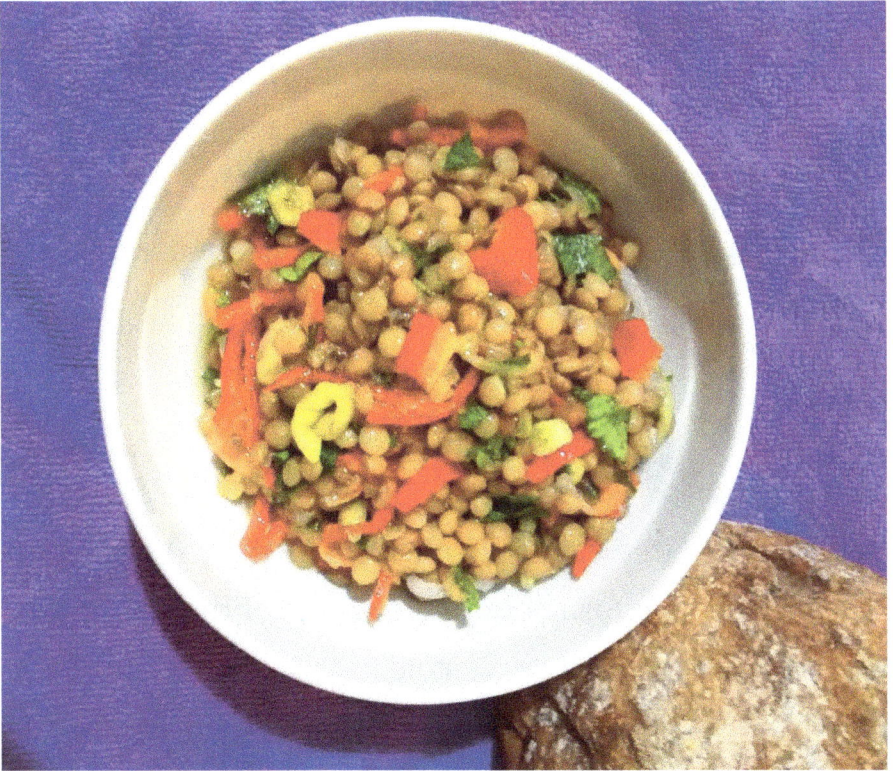

Cashews and Red Cabbage Salad

Preparation Time: 10 minutes

Cooking Time: 0 minutes

Servings: 4

Ingredients:

- 1 lb. red cabbage, shredded
- 2 tbsp. coriander, chopped
- ½ cup cashews, halved
- 2 tbsp. olive oil
- 1 tomato, cubed
- A pinch of salt and black pepper
- 1 tbsp. white vinegar

Directions:

2. In a salad bowl, combine the cabbage with the coriander and the rest of the ingredients, toss and serve cold.

Nutrition: Calories 210, Fat 6.3g, Fiber 5.2g, Carbs 5.5g, Protein 8g

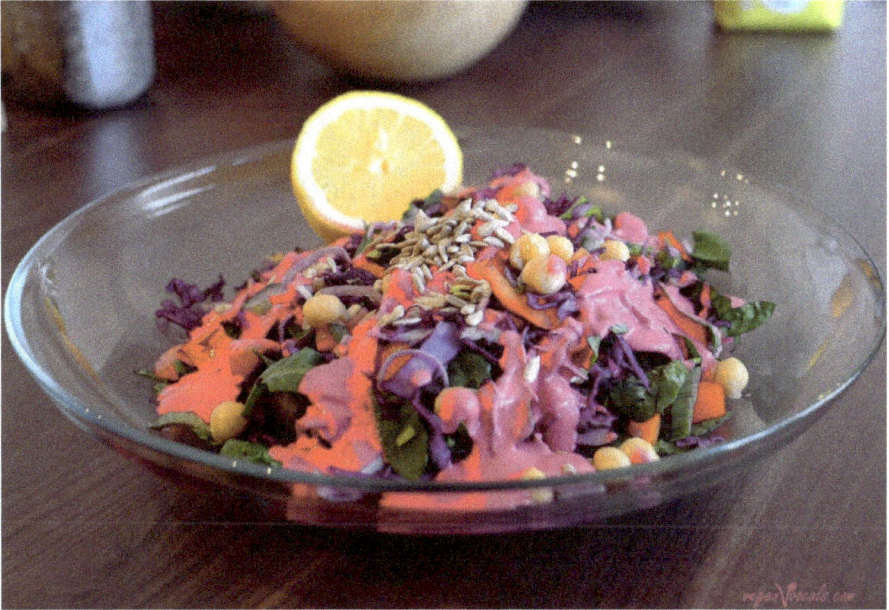

Apples and Pomegranate Salad

Preparation Time: 10 minutes

Cooking Time: 0 minutes

Servings: 4

Ingredients:

- 3 big apples, cored and cubed
- 1 cup pomegranate seeds
- 3 cups baby arugula
- 1 cup walnuts, chopped
- 1 tbsp. olive oil
- 1 tsp. white sesame seeds
- 2 tbsp. apple cider vinegar
- Salt and black pepper to the taste

Directions:

1. In a bowl, mix the apples with the arugula and the rest of the ingredients, toss and serve cold.

Nutrition: Calories 160, Fat 4.3g, Fiber 5.3g, Carbs 8.7g, Protein 10g

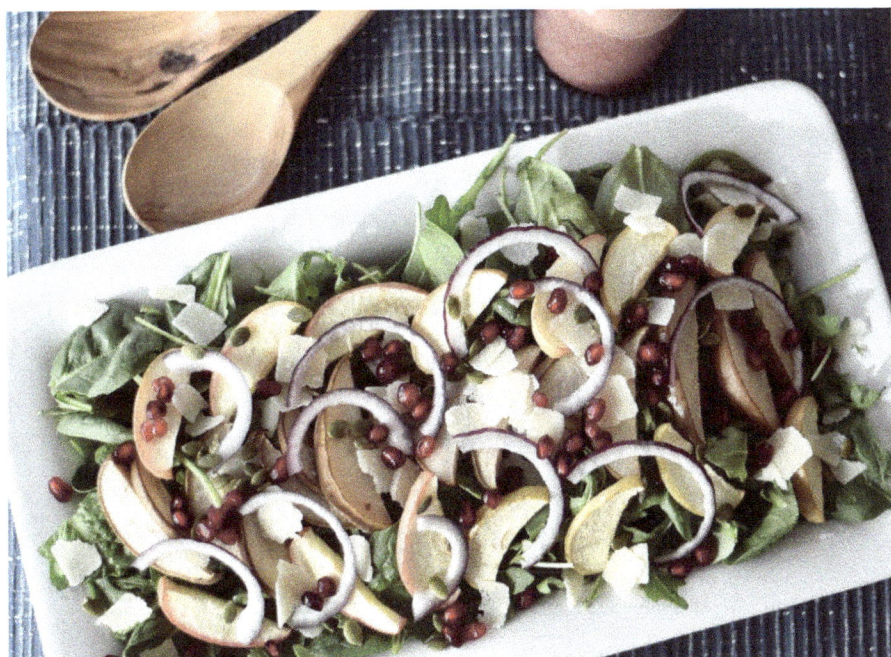

Cranberry Bulgur Mix

Preparation Time: 10 minutes

Cooking Time: 0 minutes

Servings: 4

Ingredients:

- 1 and ½ cups hot water
- 1 cup bulgur
- Juice of ½ lemon
- 4 tbsp. cilantro, chopped
- ½ cup cranberries, chopped
- 1 and ½ tsp. curry powder
- ¼ cup green onions, chopped
- ½ cup red bell peppers, chopped
- ½ cup carrots, grated
- 1 tbsp. olive oil
- A pinch of salt and black pepper

Directions:

1. Put bulgur into a bowl, add the water, stir, cover, leave aside for 10 minutes, fluff with a fork and transfer to a bowl.
2. Add the rest of the ingredients, toss, and serve cold.

Nutrition: Calories 300, Fat 6.4g, Fiber 6.1g, Carbs 7.6g, Protein 13g

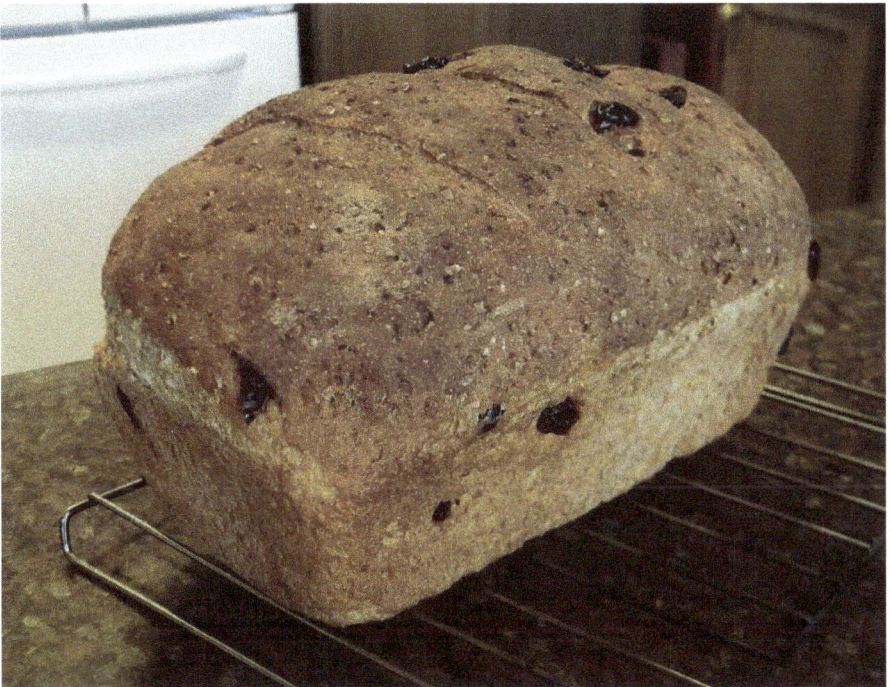

Chickpeas, Corn and Black Beans Salad

Preparation Time: 10 minutes

Cooking Time: 0 minutes

Servings: 4

Ingredients:

- 1 and ½ cups canned black beans, drained and rinsed
- ½ tsp. garlic powder
- 2 tsp. chili powder
- A pinch of sea salt and black pepper
- 1 and ½ cups canned chickpeas, drained and rinsed
- 1 cup baby spinach
- 1 avocado, pitted, peeled and chopped
- 1 cup corn kernels, chopped
- 2 tbsp. lemon juice
- 1 tbsp. olive oil
- 1 tbsp. apple cider vinegar
- 1 tsp. chives, chopped

Directions:

1. In a salad bowl, combine the black beans with the garlic powder, chili powder and the rest of the ingredients, toss and serve cold.

Nutrition: Calories 300, Fat 13.4g, Fiber 4.1g, Carbs 8.6g, Protein 13g

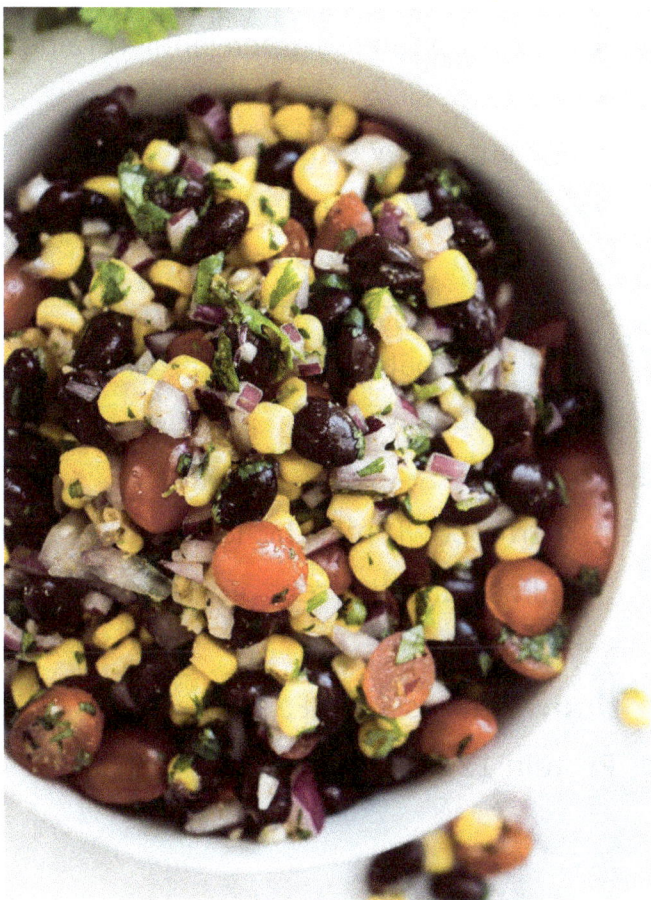

Olives and Lentils Salad

Preparation Time: 10 minutes

Cooking Time: 0 minutes

Servings: 2

Ingredients:

- 1/3 cup canned green lentils, drained and rinsed
- 1 tbsp. olive oil
- 2 cups baby spinach
- 1 cup black olives, pitted and halved
- 2 tbsp. sunflower seeds
- 1 tbsp. Dijon mustard
- 2 tbsp. balsamic vinegar
- 2 tbsp. olive oil

Directions:

1. In a bowl, mix the lentils with the spinach, olives and the rest of the ingredients, toss and serve cold.

Nutrition: Calories 279, Fat 6.5g, Fiber 4.5g, Carbs 9.6g, Protein 12g

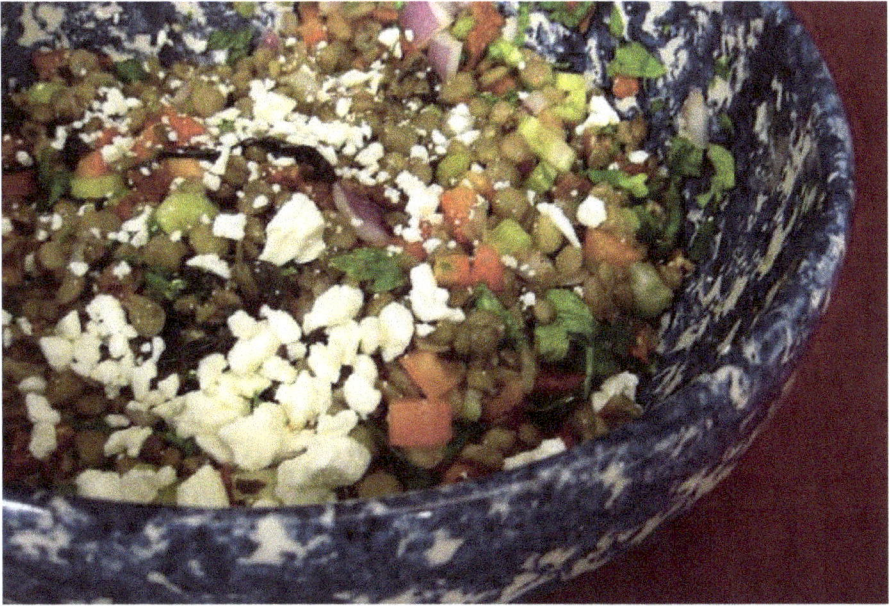

Lime Spinach and Chickpeas Salad

Preparation Time: 10 minutes

Cooking Time: 0 minutes

Servings: 4

Ingredients:

- 16 oz. canned chickpeas, drained and rinsed
- 2 cups baby spinach leaves
- ½ tbsp. lime juice
- 2 tbsp. olive oil
- 1 tsp. cumin, ground
- A pinch of sea salt and black pepper
- ½ tsp. chili flakes

Directions:

1. In a bowl, mix the chickpeas with the spinach and the rest of the ingredients, toss and serve cold.

Nutrition: Calories 240, Fat 8.2g, Fiber 5.3g, Carbs 11.6g, Protein 12g

Beans and Cucumber Salad

Preparation Time: 10 minutes

Cooking Time: 0 minutes

Servings: 4

Ingredients:

- 15 oz. canned great northern beans, drained and rinsed
- 2 tbsp. olive oil
- ½ cup baby arugula
- 1 cup cucumber, sliced
- 1 tbsp. parsley, chopped
- 2 tomatoes, cubed
- A pinch of sea salt and black pepper
- 2 tbsp. balsamic vinegar

Directions:

2. In a bowl, mix the beans with the cucumber and the rest of the ingredients, toss and serve cold.

Nutrition: Calories 233, Fat 9g, Fiber 6.5g, Carbs 13g, Protein 8g

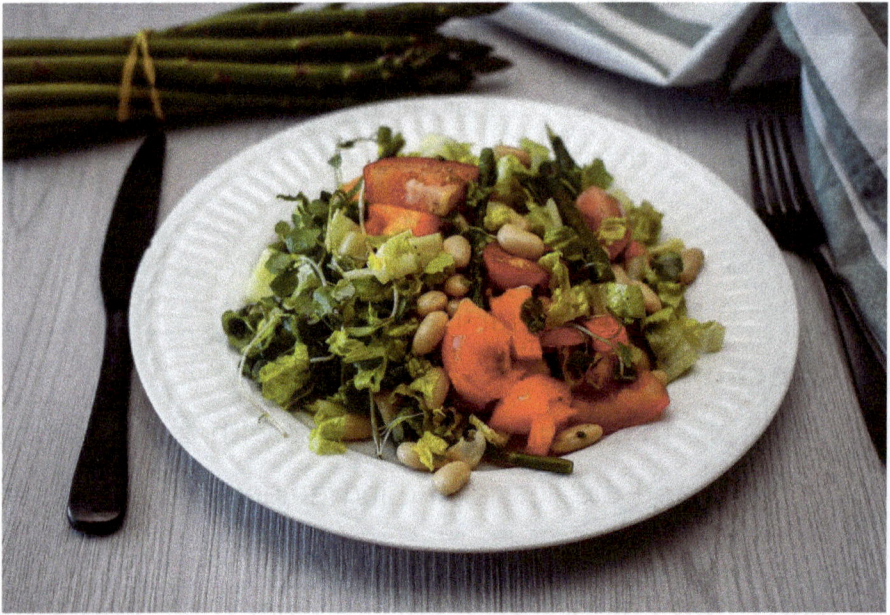

Minty Olives and Tomatoes Salad

Preparation Time: 10 minutes

Cooking Time: 0 minutes

Servings: 4

Ingredients:

- 1 cup kalamata olives, pitted and sliced
- 1 cup black olives, pitted and halved
- 1 cup cherry tomatoes, halved
- 4 tomatoes, chopped
- 1 red onion, chopped
- 2 tbsp. oregano, chopped
- 1 tbsp. mint, chopped
- 2 tbsp. balsamic vinegar
- ¼ cup olive oil
- 2 tsp. Italian herbs, dried
- A pinch of sea salt and black pepper

Directions:

1. In a salad bowl, mix the olives with the tomatoes and the rest of the ingredients, toss and serve cold.

Nutrition: Calories 190, Fat 8.1g, Fiber 5.8g, Carbs 11.6g, Protein 4.6g

Tomato And Avocado Salad

Preparation Time: 10 minutes

Cooking Time: 0 minutes

Servings: 4

Ingredients:

- 1 lb. cherry tomatoes, cubed
- 2 avocados, pitted, peeled and cubed
- 1 sweet onion, chopped
- A pinch of sea salt and black pepper
- 2 tbsp. lemon juice
- 1 and ½ tbsp. olive oil
- A handful basil, chopped

Directions:

1. In a salad bowl, mix the tomatoes with the avocados and the rest of the ingredients, toss and serve right away.

Nutrition: Calories 148, Fat 7.8g, Fiber 2.9g, Carbs 5.4g, Protein 5.5g

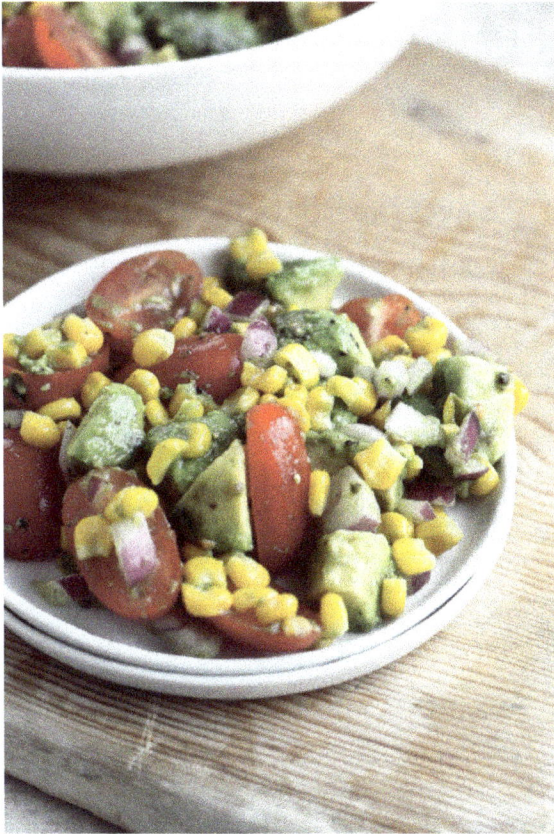

Corn and Tomato Salad

Preparation Time: 10 minutes

Cooking Time: 0 minutes

Servings: 4

Ingredients:

- 2 avocados, pitted, peeled and cubed
- 1 pint mixed cherry tomatoes, halved:
- 2 tbsp. avocado oil
- 1 tbsp. lime juice
- ½ tsp. lime zest, grated
- A pinch of salt and black pepper
- ¼ cup dill, chopped

Directions:

1. In a salad bowl, mix the avocados with the tomatoes and the rest of the ingredients, toss and serve cold.

Nutrition: Calories 188, Fat 7.3g, Fiber 4.9g, Carbs 6.4g, Protein 6.5g

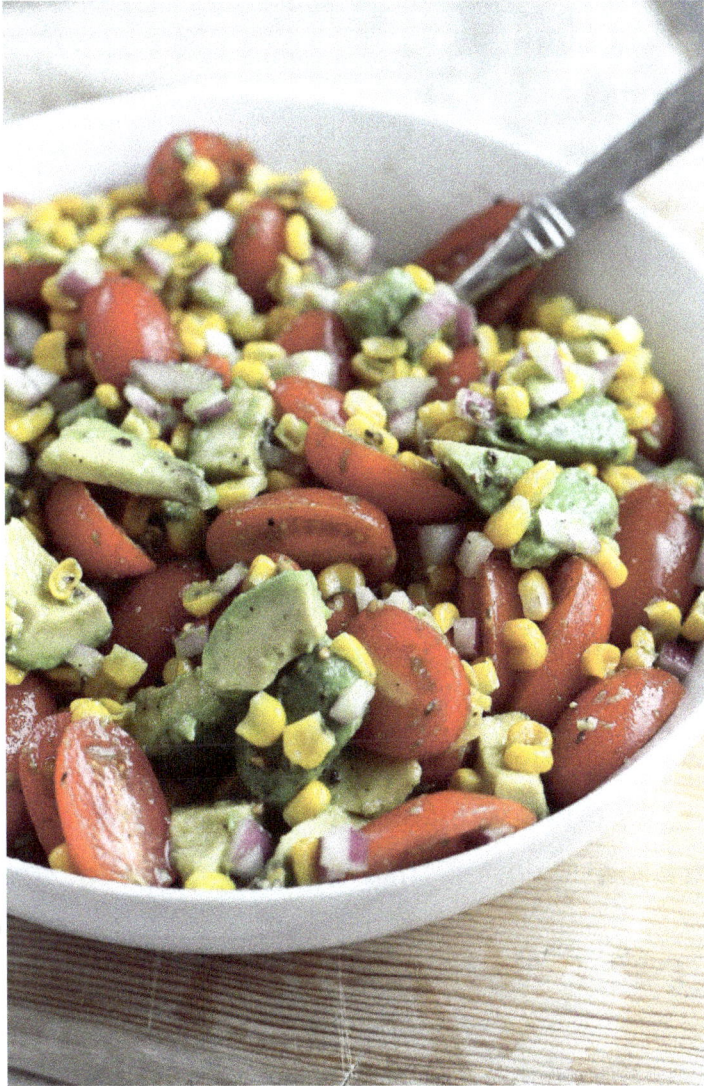

Orange and Cucumber Salad

Preparation Time: 10 minutes

Cooking Time: 0 minutes

Servings: 4

Ingredients:

- 2 cucumbers, sliced
- 1 orange, peeled and cut into segments
- 1 cup cherry tomatoes, halved
- 1 small red onion, chopped
- 3 tbsp. olive oil
- 4 and ½ tsp. balsamic vinegar
- Salt and black pepper to the taste
- 1 tbsp. lemon juice

Directions:

1. In a bowl, mix the cucumbers with the orange and the rest of the ingredients, toss and serve cold.

Nutrition: Calories 102, Fat 7.5g, Fiber 3g, Carbs 6.1g, Protein 3.4g

Parsley and Corn Salad

Preparation Time: 10 minutes

Cooking Time: 0 minutes

Servings: 4

Ingredients:

- 1 and ½ tsp. balsamic vinegar
- 2 tbsp. lime juice
- 2 tbsp. olive oil
- A pinch of sea salt and black pepper
- Black pepper to the taste
- 4 cups corn
- ½ cup parsley, chopped
- 2 spring onions, chopped

Directions:

1. In a salad bowl, combine the corn with the onions and the rest of the ingredients, toss and serve cold.

Nutrition: Calories 121, Fat 9.5g, Fiber 1.8g, Carbs 4.1g, Protein 1.9g

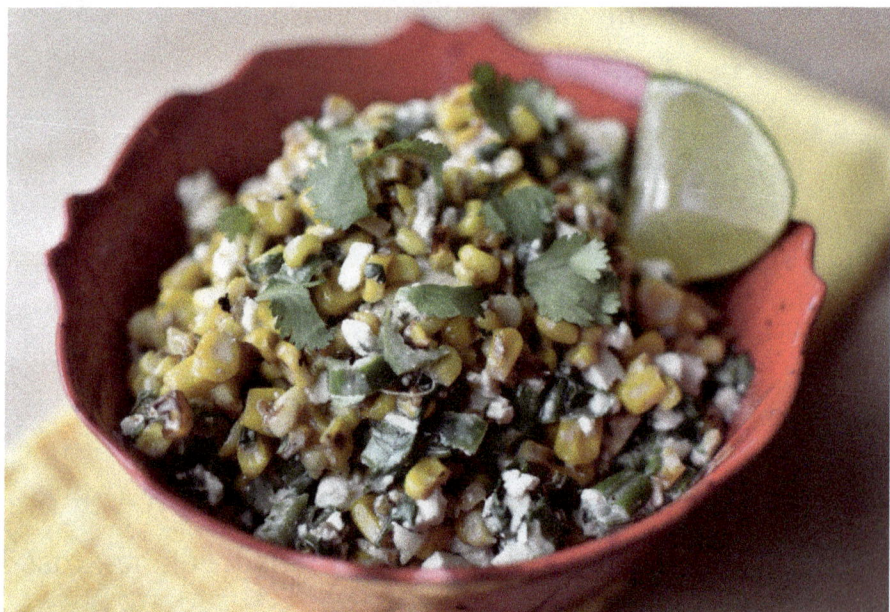

Radish and Corn Salad

Preparation Time: 10 minutes

Cooking Time: 0 minutes

Servings: 2

Ingredients:

- 1 tbsp. lemon juice
- 1 jalapeno, chopped
- 2 tbsp. olive oil
- ¼ tsp. oregano, dried
- A pinch of sea salt and black pepper
- 2 cups fresh corn
- 6 radishes, sliced

Directions:

1. In a salad bowl, combine the corn with the radishes and the rest of the ingredients, toss and serve cold.

Nutrition: Calories 134, Fat 4.5g, Fiber 1.8g, Carbs 4.1g, Protein 1.9g

Arugula and Corn Salad

Preparation Time: 10 minutes

Cooking Time: 0 minutes

Servings: 4

Ingredients:

- 1 red bell pepper, thinly sliced
- 2 cups corn
- Juice of 1 lime
- Zest of 1 lime, grated
- 8 cups baby arugula
- A pinch of sea salt and black pepper

Directions:

1. In a salad bowl, mix the corn with the arugula and the rest of the ingredients, toss and serve cold.

Nutrition: Calories 172, Fat 8.5g, Fiber 1.8g, Carbs 5.1g, Protein 1.4g

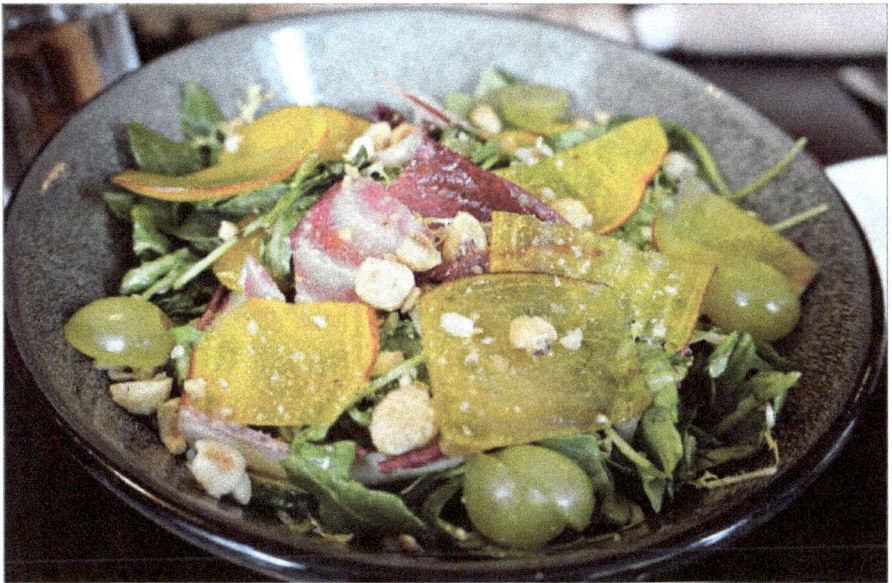

Balsamic Bulgur Salad

Preparation Time: 30 minutes

Cooking Time: 0 minutes

Servings: 4

Ingredients:

- 1 cup bulgur
- 2 cups hot water
- 1 cucumber, sliced
- A pinch of sea salt and black pepper
- 2 tbsp. lemon juice
- 2 tbsp. balsamic vinegar
- ¼ cup olive oil

Directions:

1. In a bowl, mix bulgur with the water, cover, leave aside for 30 minutes, fluff with a fork and transfer to a salad bowl.

Add the rest of the ingredients, toss and serve.

Nutrition: Calories 171, Fat 5.1g, Fiber 6.1g, Carbs 11.3g, Protein 4.4g

Healthy Coconut Blueberry Balls

Preparation Time: 10 minutes

Cooking Time: 10 minutes

Servings: 12

Ingredients:

- ¼ cup flaked coconut
- ¼ cup blueberries
- ½ tsp. vanilla
- ¼ cup honey
- ½ cup creamy almond butter
- ¼ tsp. cinnamon
- 1 ½ tbsp. chia seeds
- ¼ cup flaxseed meal
- 1 cup rolled oats, gluten-free

Directions:

1. In a large bowl, add oats, cinnamon, chia seeds, and flaxseed meal and mix well.
2. Add almond butter in microwave-safe bowl and microwave for 30 seconds. Stir until smooth.

3.   Add vanilla and honey in melted almond butter and stir well.
4.   Pour almond butter mixture over oat mixture and stir to combine.
5.   Add coconut and blueberries and stir well.
6.   Make small balls from oat mixture and place onto the baking tray and place in the refrigerator for 1 hour.
7.   Serve and enjoy.

Nutrition:

Calories 129,

Fat 7.4g,

Carbs 14.1g,

Sugar 7g,

Protein 4 g,

Cholesterol 0 mg

Crunchy Roasted Chickpeas

Preparation Time: 10 minutes

Cooking Time: 25 minutes

Servings: 4

Ingredients:

- 15 oz can chickpeas, drained, rinsed and pat dry
- ¼ tsp. paprika
- 1 tbsp. olive oil
- ¼ tsp. pepper
- Pinch of salt

Directions:

1. Preheat the oven to 450°F.
2. Spray a baking tray with cooking spray and set aside.
3. In a large bowl, toss chickpeas with olive oil and spread chickpeas onto the prepared baking tray.
4. Roast chickpeas in preheated oven for 25 minutes. Shake after every 10 minutes.
5. Once chickpeas are done then immediately toss with paprika, pepper, and salt.
6. Serve and enjoy.

Nutrition:

Calories 157,

Fat 4.7g,

Carbs 24.2g,

Protein 5.3g,

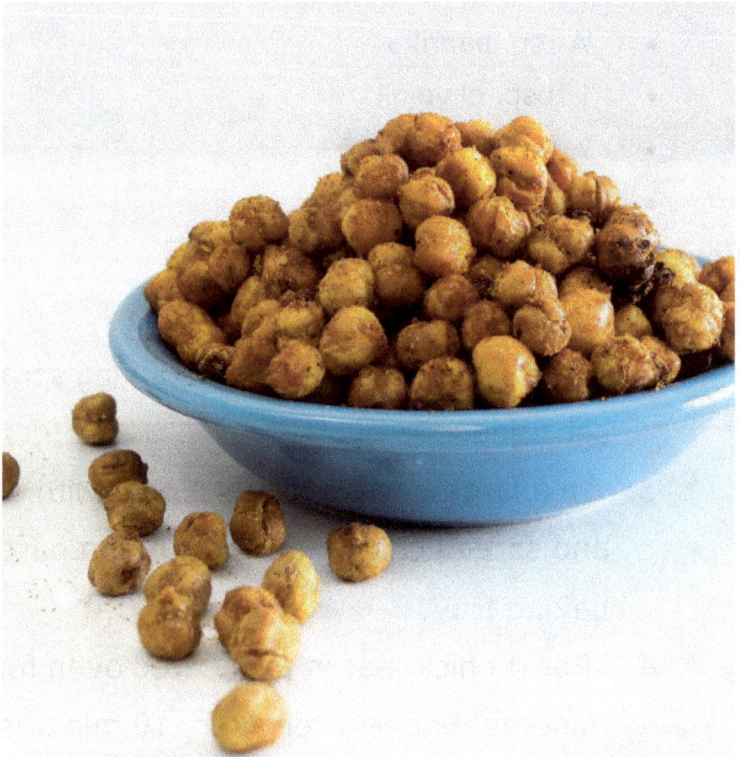

Tasty Zucchini Chips

Preparation Time: 10 minutes

Cooking Time: 15 minutes

Servings: 8

Ingredients:

- 2 medium zucchini, sliced 4mm thick
- ½ tsp. paprika
- ¼ tsp. garlic powder
- ¾ cup parmesan cheese, grated
- 4 tbsp. olive oil
- ¼ tsp. pepper
- Pinch of salt

Directions:

1. Preheat the oven to 375°F.
2. Spray a baking tray with cooking spray and set aside.
3. In a bowl, combine the oil, garlic powder, paprika, pepper, and salt.
4. Add sliced zucchini and toss to coat.
5. Arrange zucchini slices onto the prepared baking tray and sprinkle grated cheese on top.
6. Bake in preheated oven for 15 minutes or until lightly golden brown.
7. Serve and enjoy.

Nutrition:

Calories 110,

Fat 9.8g,

Carbs 2.2g,

Protein 4.4g

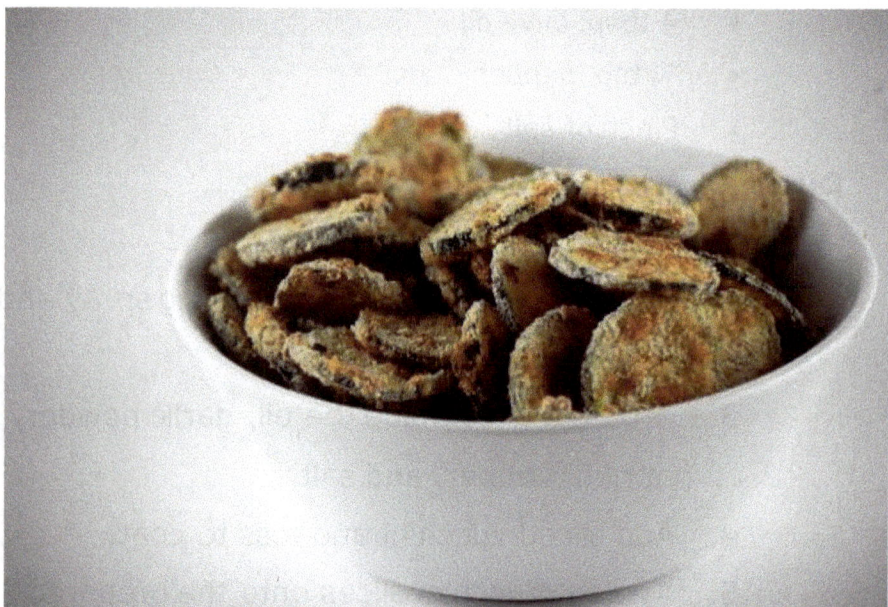

Roasted Green Beans

Preparation Time: 10 minutes

Cooking Time: 15 minutes

Servings: 4

Ingredients:

- 1 lb green beans
- 4 tbsp. parmesan cheese
- 2 tbsp. olive oil
- ¼ tsp. garlic powder
- Pinch of salt

Directions:

1. Preheat the oven to 400°F.
2. Add green beans in a large bowl.
3. Add remaining ingredients on top of green beans and toss to coat.
4. Spread green beans onto the baking tray and roast in preheated oven for 15 minutes. Stir halfway through.
5. Serve and enjoy.

Nutrition:

Calories 101,

Fat 7.5g,

Carbs 8.3g,

Sugar 1.6g,

Protein 2.6g,

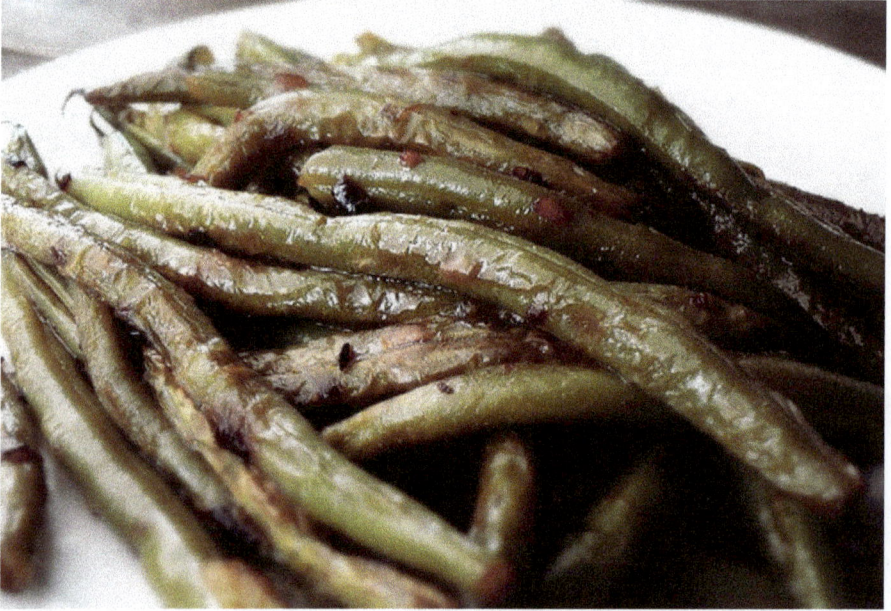

Savory Pistachio Balls

Preparation Time: 10 minutes

Cooking Time: 5 minutes

Servings: 16

Ingredients:

- ½ cup pistachios, unsalted
- 1 cup dates, pitted
- ½ tsp. ground fennel seeds
- ½ cup raisins
- Pinch of pepper

Directions:

1. Add all ingredients into the food processor and process until well combined.
2. Make small balls and place onto the baking tray and place in the refrigerator for 1 hour.
3. Serve and enjoy.

Nutrition:

Calories 55,

Fat 0.9g,

Carbs 12.5g,

Sugar 9.9g,

Protein 0.8g,

Cholesterol 0mg

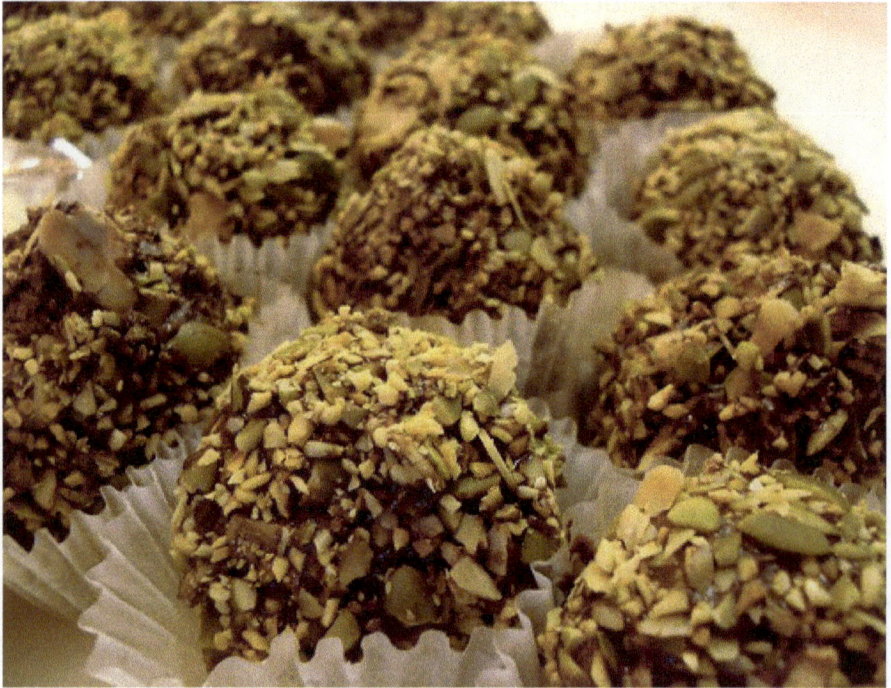

Roasted Almonds

Preparation Time: 10 minutes

Cooking Time: 20 minutes

Servings: 12

Ingredients :

- 2 ½ cups almonds
- ¼ tsp. cayenne
- ¼ tsp. ground coriander
- ¼ tsp. cumin
- ¼ tsp. chili powder
- 1 tbsp. fresh rosemary, chopped
- 1 tbsp. olive oil
- 2 ½ tbsp. maple syrup
- Pinch of salt

Directions:

1. Preheat the oven to 325°F.

2. Spray a baking tray with cooking spray and set aside.

3. In a mixing bowl, whisk together oil, cayenne, coriander, cumin, chili powder, rosemary, maple syrup, and salt.

4. Add almond and stir to coat.

5. Spread almonds onto the prepared baking tray.

6. Roast almonds in preheated oven for 20 minutes. Stir halfway through.

7. Serve and enjoy.

Nutrition:

Calories 137,

Fat 11.2g,

Carbs 7.3g,

Protein 4.2g,

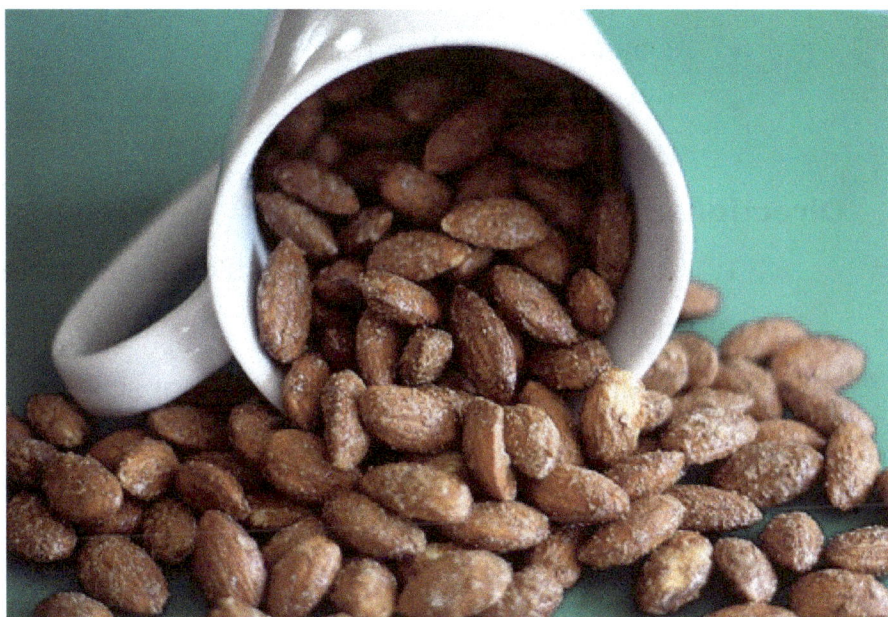

Banana Strawberry Popsicles

Preparation Time: 5 minutes

Cooking Time: 0 minutes

Servings: 8

Ingredients :

- ½ cup Greek yogurt
- 1 banana, peeled and sliced
- 1 ¼ cup fresh strawberries
- ¼ cup of water

Directions:

1. Add all ingredients into the blender and blend until smooth.
2. Pour blended mixture into the popsicles molds and place in the refrigerator for 4 hours or until set.
3. Serve and enjoy.

Nutrition:

Calories 31,

Fat 0. g,

Carbs 6.2g,

Protein 1.2g ,

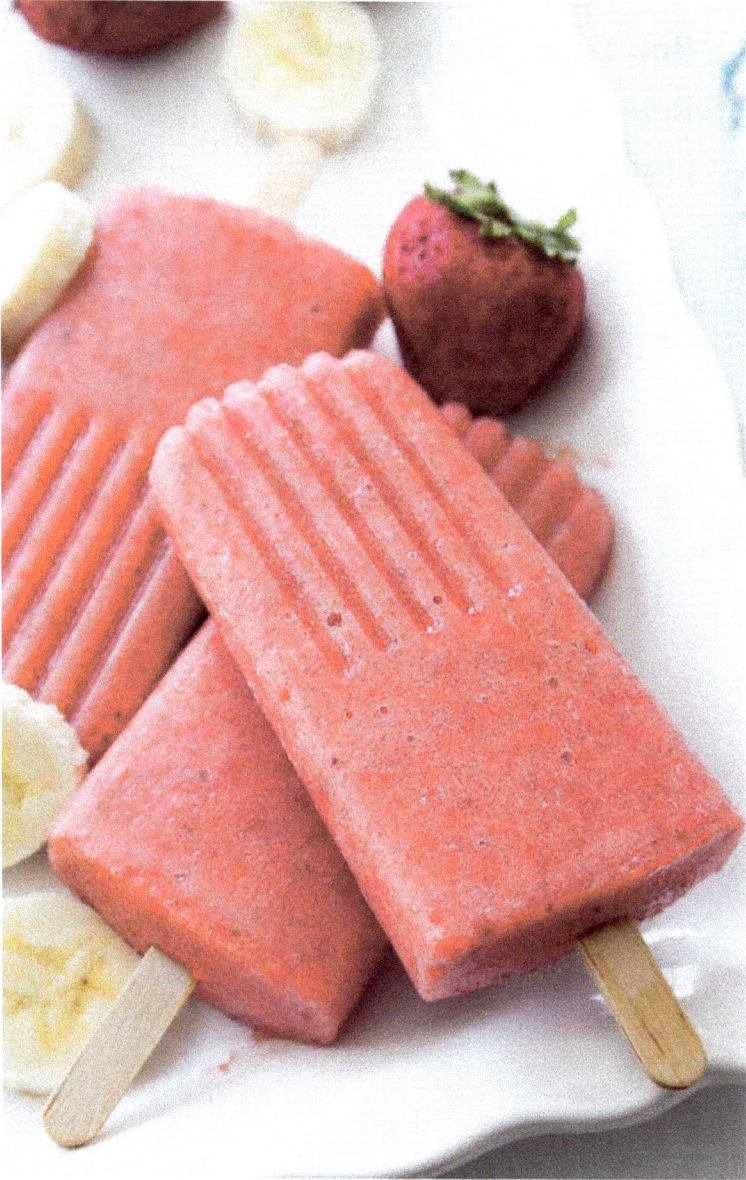

Chocolate Matcha Balls

Preparation Time: 10 minutes

Cooking Time: 5 minutes

Servings: 15

Ingredients:

- 2 tbsp. unsweetened cocoa powder
- 3 tbsp. oats, gluten-free
- ½ cup pine nuts
- ½ cup almonds
- 1 cup dates, pitted
- 2 tbsp. matcha powder

Directions:

1. Add oats, pine nuts, almonds, and dates into a food processor and process until well combined.
2. Place matcha powder in a small dish.
3. Make small balls from mixture and coat with matcha powder.
4. Enjoy or store in refrigerator until ready to eat.

Nutrition:

Calories 88,

Fat 4.9g,

Carbs 11.3g,

Protein 1.9g

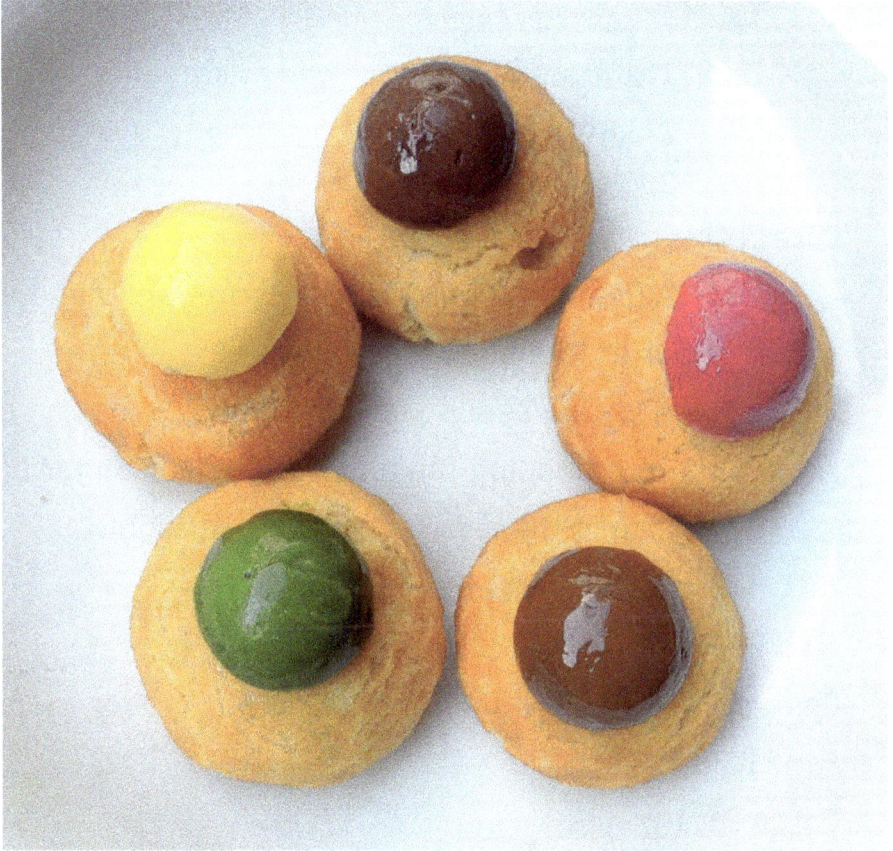

Chia Almond Butter Pudding

Preparation Time: 5 minutes

Cooking Time: 5 minutes

Servings: 1

Ingredients:

- ¼ cup chia seeds
- 1 cup unsweetened almond milk
- 1 ½ tbsp. maple syrup
- 2 ½ tbsp. almond butter

Directions:

1. Add almond milk, maple syrup, and almond butter in a bowl and stir well.
2. Add chia seeds and stir to mix.
3. Pour pudding mixture into the Mason jar and place in the refrigerator for overnight.
4. Serve and enjoy.

Nutrition:

Calories 354,

Fat 21.3g,

Carbs 31.1g,

Protein 11.2g,

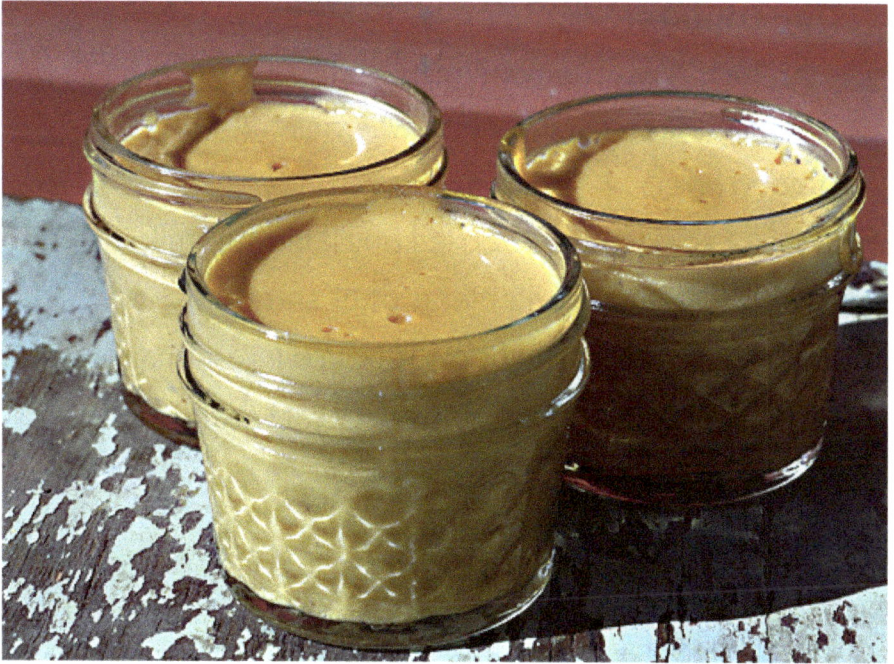

Refreshing Strawberry Popsicles

Preparation Time: 5 minutes

Cooking Time: 5 minutes

Servings: 8

Ingredients:

- ½ cup almond milk
- 2 ½ cup fresh strawberries

Directions:

1. Add strawberries and almond milk into the blender and blend until smooth.
2. Pour strawberry mixture into popsicles molds and place in the refrigerator for 4 hours or until set.
3. Serve and enjoy.

Nutrition:

Calories 49,

Fat 3.7g,

Carbs 4.3g,

Protein 0.6g,

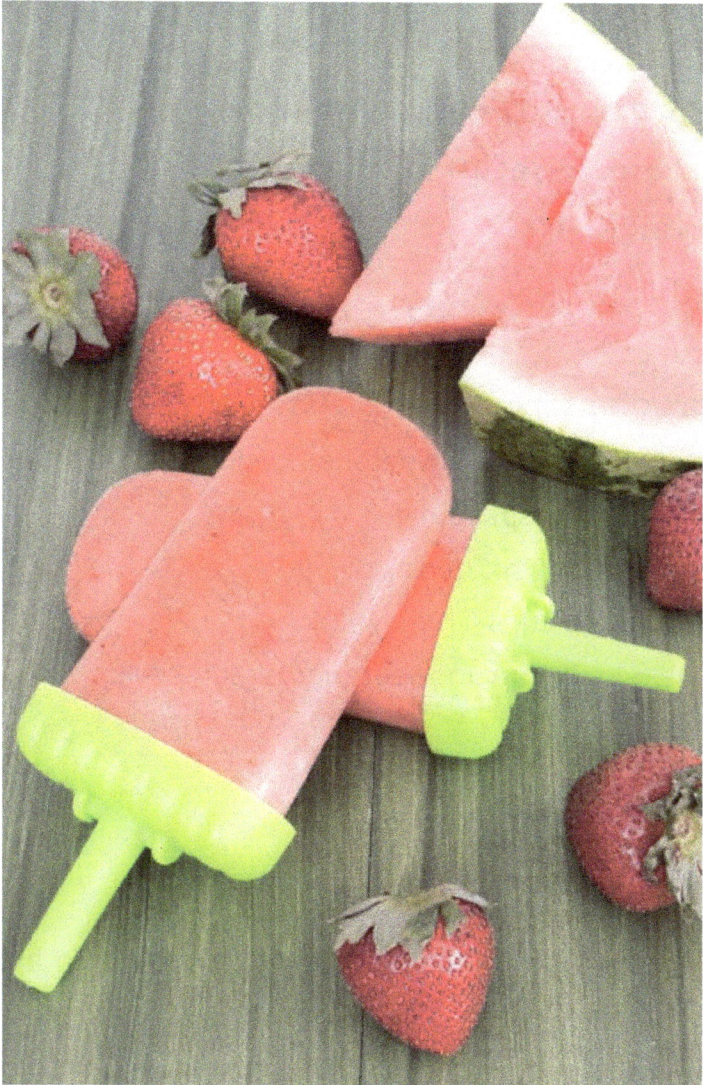

Dark Chocolate Mousse

Preparation Time: 10 minutes

Cooking Time: 10 minutes

Servings: 4

Ingredients:

- 3.5oz unsweetened dark chocolate, grated
- ½ tsp. vanilla
- 1 tbsp. honey
- 2 cups Greek yogurt
- ¾ cup unsweetened almond milk

Directions:

1. Add chocolate and almond milk in a saucepan and heat over medium heat until just chocolate melted. Do not boil.

2. Once the chocolate and almond milk combined then add vanilla and honey and stir well.
3. Add yogurt in a large mixing bowl.
4. Pour chocolate mixture on top of yogurt and mix until well combined.
5. Pour chocolate yogurt mixture into the serving bowls and place in refrigerator for 2 hours.
6. Top with fresh raspberries and serve.

Nutrition:

Calories 278,

Fat 15.4g,

Carbs 20g,

Protein 10.5g,

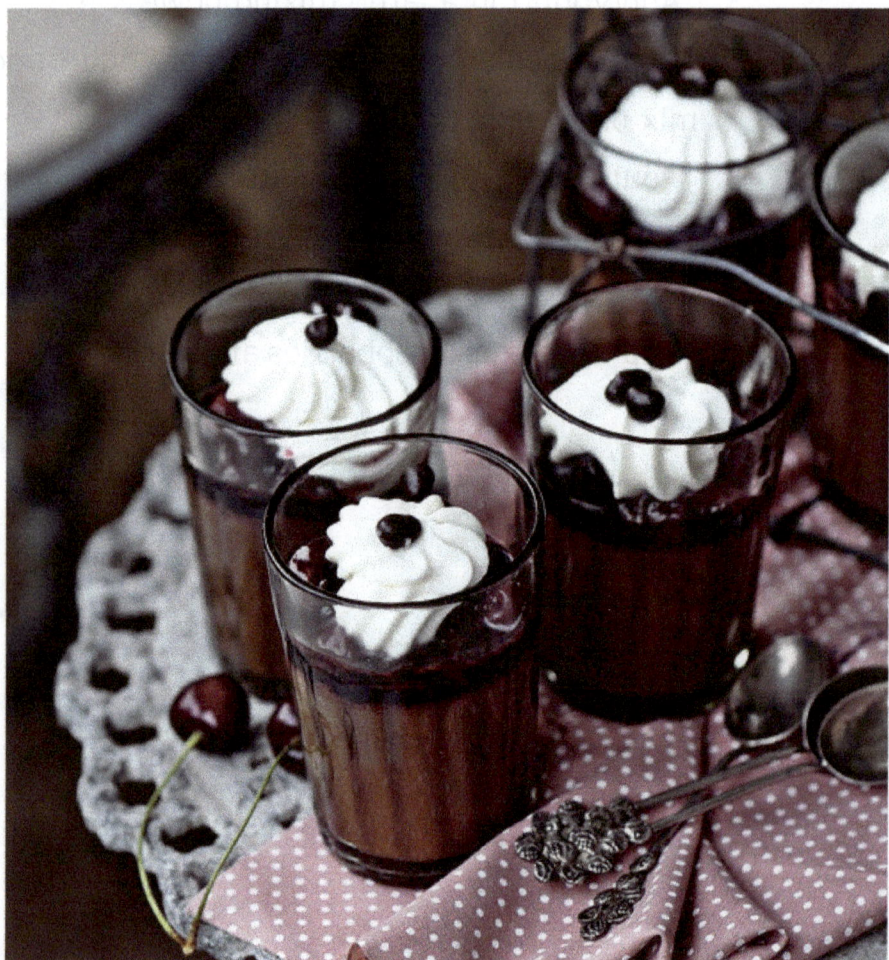

Warm & Soft Baked Pears

Preparation Time: 10 minutes

Cooking Time: 25 minutes

Servings: 4

Ingredients:

- 4 pears, cut in half and core
- ½ tsp. vanilla
- ¼ tsp. cinnamon
- ½ cup maple syrup

Directions:

1. Preheat the oven to 375°F.
2. Spray a baking tray with cooking spray.
3. Arrange pears, cut side up on a prepared baking tray and sprinkle with cinnamon.
4. In a small bowl, whisk vanilla and maple syrup and drizzle over pears.
5. Bake pears in preheated oven for 25 minutes.
6. Serve and enjoy.

Nutrition:

Calories 226,

Fat 0.4g,

Carbs 58.4g,

Sugar 43.9g,

Protein 0.8g,

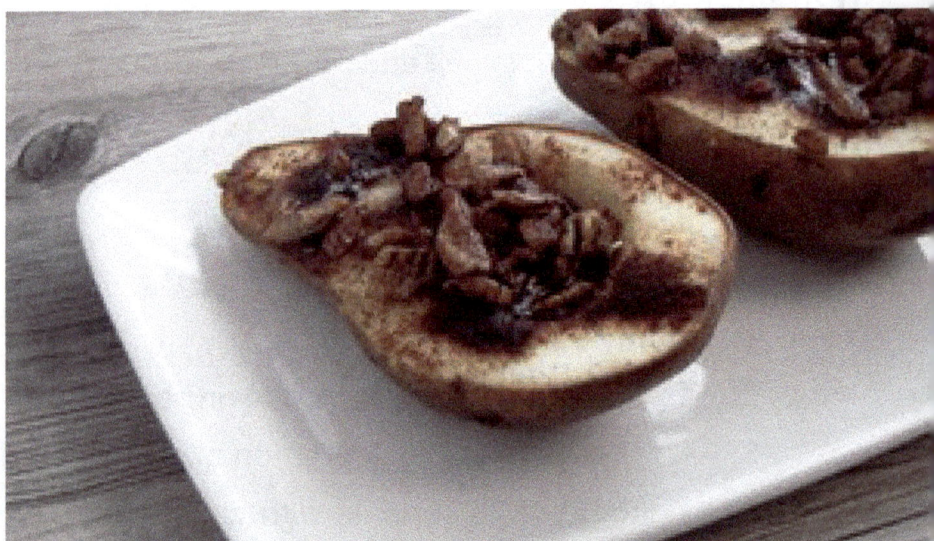

Healthy & Quick Energy Bites

Preparation Time: 10 minutes

Cooking Time: 0 minutes

Servings: 20

Ingredients:

- 2 cups cashew nuts
- ¼ tsp. cinnamon
- 1 tsp. lemon zest
- 4 tbsp. dates, chopped
- 1/3 cup unsweetened shredded coconut
- ¾ cup dried apricots

Directions:

1. Line baking tray with parchment paper and set aside.
2. Add all ingredients in a food processor and process until the mixture is crumbly and well combined.
3. Make small balls from mixture and place on a prepared baking tray.
4. Place in refrigerator for 1 hour.
5. Serve and enjoy.

Nutrition:

Calories 100,

Fat 7.5g,

Carbs 7.2g,

Protein 2.4g,

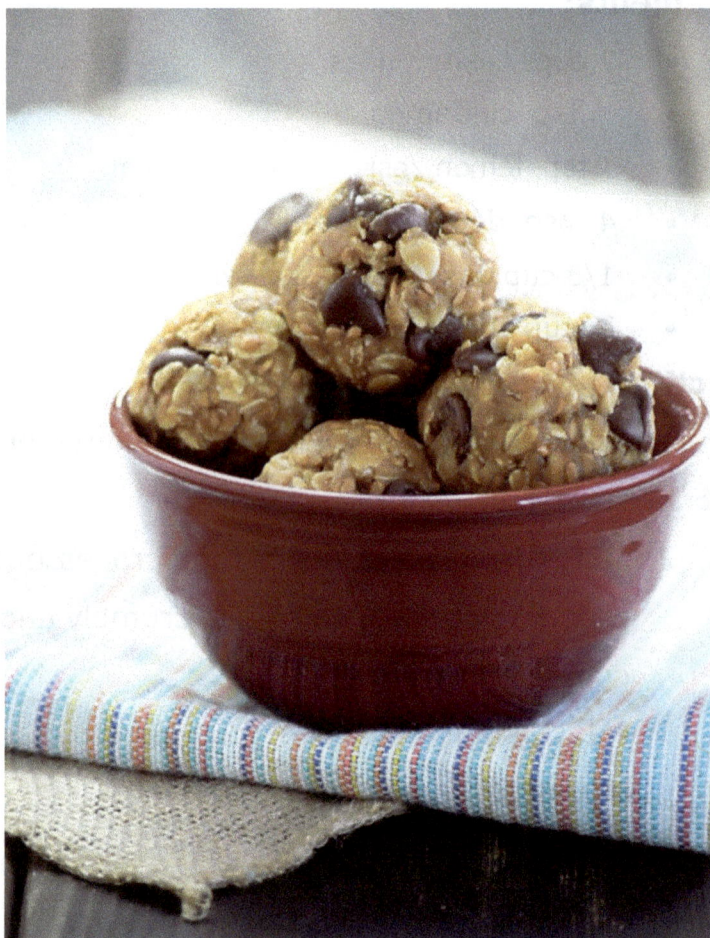

Creamy Yogurt Banana Bowls

Preparation Time: 10 minutes

Cooking Time: 0 minutes

Servings: 4

Ingredients:

- 2 bananas, sliced
- ½ tsp. ground nutmeg
- 3 tbsp. flaxseed meal
- ¼ cup creamy peanut butter
- 4 cups Greek yogurt

Directions:

1. Divide Greek yogurt between 4 serving bowls and top with sliced bananas.
2. Add peanut butter in microwave-safe bowl and microwave for 30 seconds.
3. Drizzle 1 tbsp. of melted peanut butter on each bowl on top of the sliced bananas.
4. Sprinkle cinnamon and flax meal on top and serve.

Nutrition:

Calories 351,

Fat 13.1g,

Carbs 35.6g, ,

Protein 19.6g,

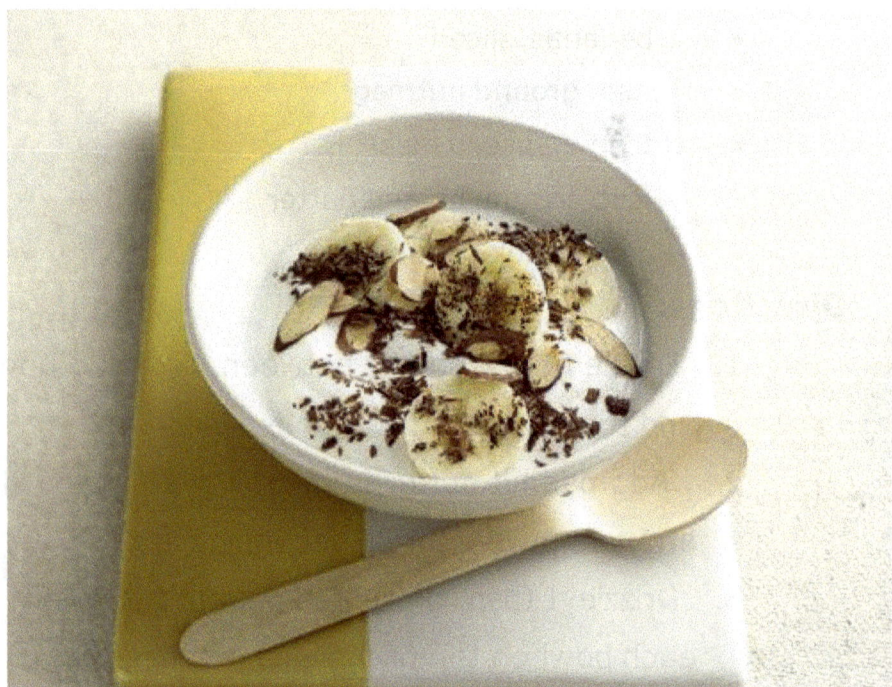

Chicken Wings Platter

Preparation Time: 10 minutes

Cooking Time: 20 minutes

Serves: 4

Ingredients:

- 2 lb. chicken wings
- ½ cup tomato sauce
- A pinch of salt and black pepper
- 1 tsp. smoked paprika
- 1 tbsp. cilantro, chopped
- 1 tbsp. chives, chopped

Directions:

1. In your instant pot, combine the chicken wings with the sauce and the rest of the ingredients, stir, put the lid on and cook on High for 20 minutes.
2. Release the pressure naturally for 10 minutes, arrange the chicken wings on a platter and serve as an appetizer.

Nutrition:

Calories 203,

Fat 13g,

Fiber 3g,

Carbs 5g,

Protein 8g

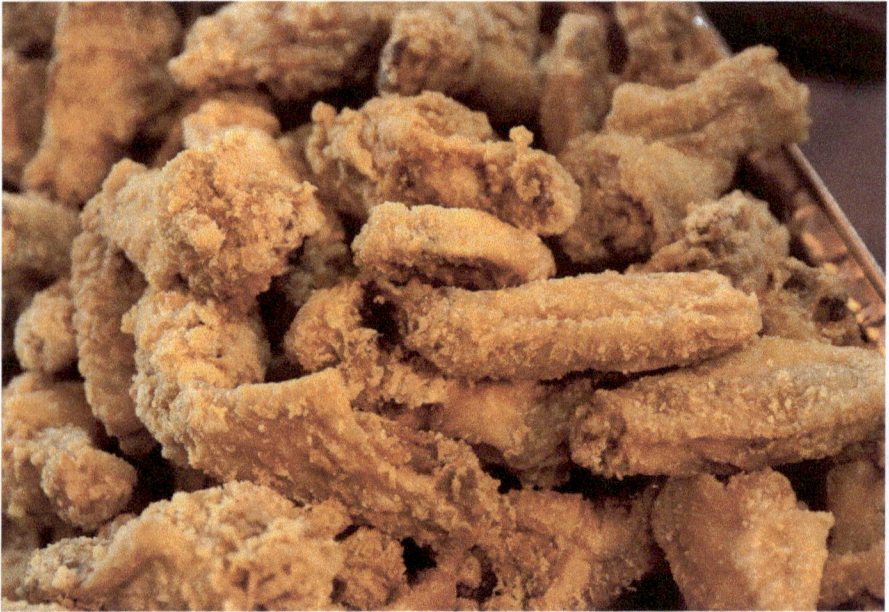

Carrot Spread

Preparation Time: 10 minutes

Cooking Time: 10 minutes

Serves: 4

Ingredients:

- ¼ cup veggie stock
- A pinch of salt and black pepper
- 1 tsp. onion powder
- ½ tsp. garlic powder
- ½ tsp. oregano, dried
- 1 lb. carrots, sliced
- ½ cup coconut cream

Directions:

1. In your instant pot, combine all the ingredients except the cream, put the lid on and cook on High for 10 minutes.
2. Release the pressure naturally for 10 minutes, transfer the carrots mix to food processor, add the cream, pulse well, divide into bowls and serve cold.

Nutrition:

Calories 124,

Fat 1g,

Fiber 2g,

Carbs 5g,

Protein 8g

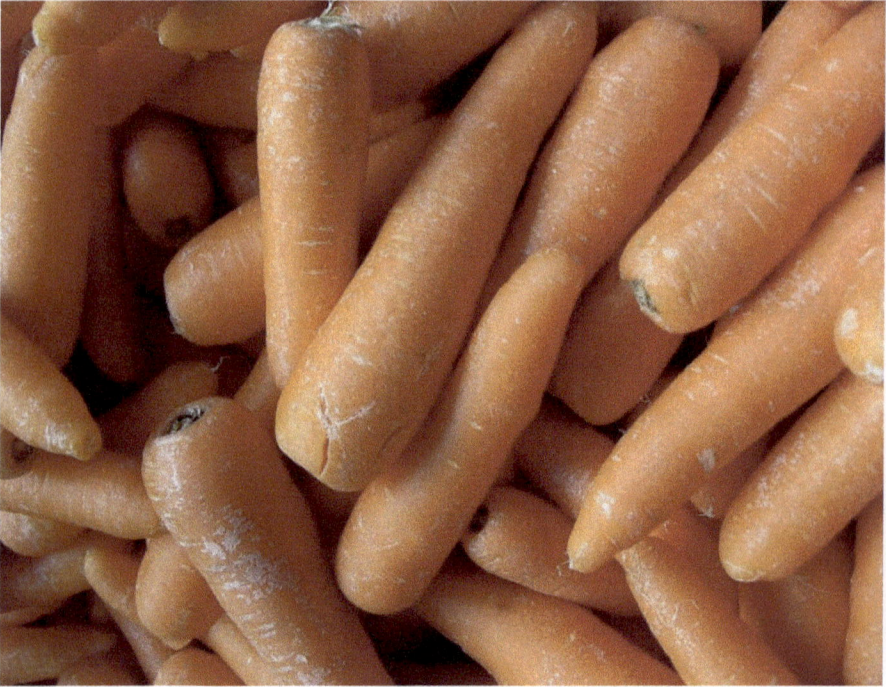

Chocolate Mousse

Preparation Time: 10 minutes

Cooking Time: 6 minutes

Servings: 5

Ingredients:

- 4 egg yolks
- ½ tsp. vanilla
- ½ cup unsweetened almond milk
- 1 cup whipping cream
- ¼ cup cocoa powder
- ¼ cup water
- ½ cup Swerve
- 1/8 tsp. salt

Directions:

1. Add egg yolks to a large bowl and whisk until well beaten.
2. In a saucepan, add swerve, cocoa powder, and water and whisk until well combined.
3. Add almond milk and cream to the saucepan and whisk until well mix.
4. Once saucepan mixtures are heated up then turn off the heat.
5. Add vanilla and salt and stir well.
6. Add a tbsp. of chocolate mixture into the eggs and whisk until well combined.

7. Slowly pour remaining chocolate to the eggs and whisk until well combined.
8. Pour batter into the ramekins.
9. Pour 1 ½ cups of water into the instant pot then place a trivet in the pot.
10. Place ramekins on a trivet.
11. Seal pot with lid and select manual and set timer for 6 minutes.
12. Release pressure using quick release method than open the lid.
13. Carefully remove ramekins from the instant pot and let them cool completely.
14. Serve and enjoy.

Nutrition:

Calories 128,

Fat 11.9g,

Carbs 4g,

Protein 3.6g

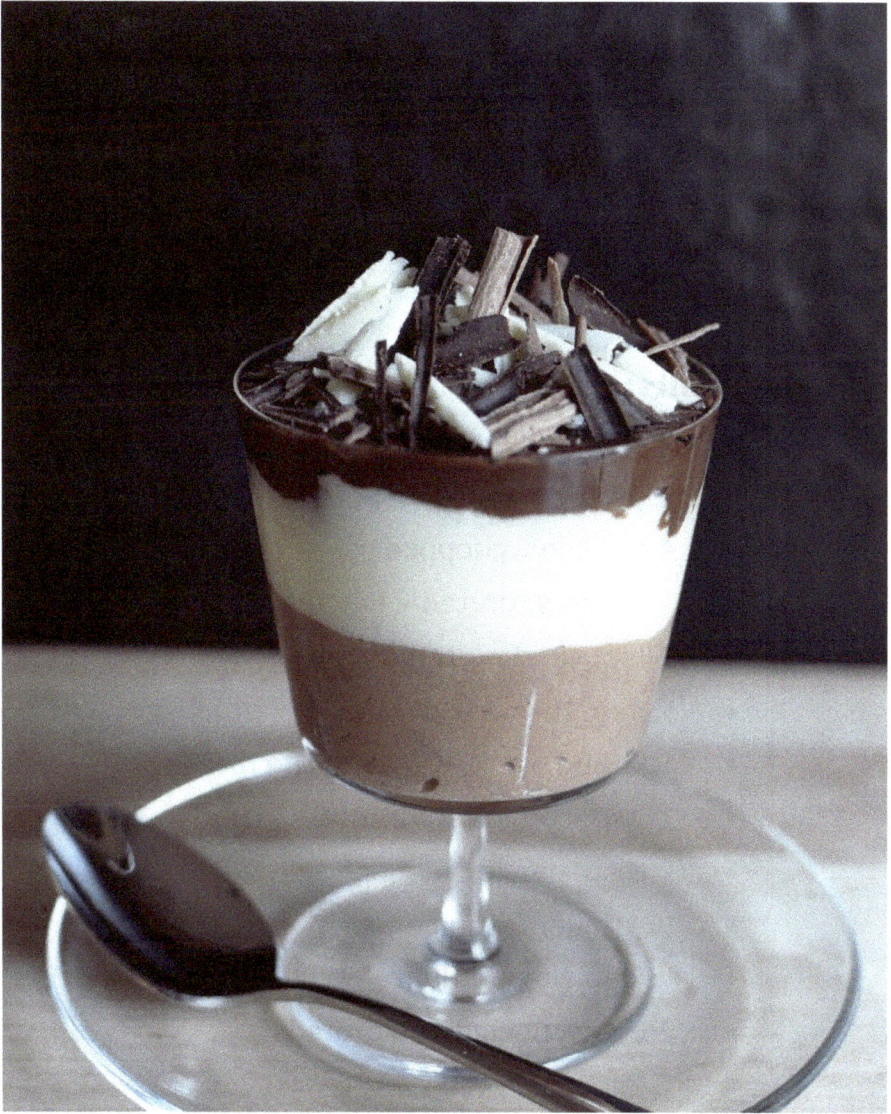

Veggie Fritters

Preparation Time: 10 minutes
Cooking Time: 10 minutes
Servings: 4

Ingredients:

- 2 garlic cloves, minced
- 2 yellow onions, chopped
- 4 scallions, chopped
- 2 carrots, grated
- 2 tsp. cumin, ground
- ½ tsp. turmeric powder
- Salt and black pepper to the taste
- ¼ tsp. coriander, ground
- 2 tbsp. parsley, chopped
- ¼ tsp. lemon juice
- ½ cup almond flour
- 2 beets, peeled and grated
- 2 eggs, whisked
- ¼ cup tapioca flour
- 3 tbsp. olive oil

Directions:

1. In a bowl, combine the garlic with the onions, scallions and the rest of the ingredients except the oil, stir well and shape medium fritters out of this mix.

2. Heat up a pan with the oil over medium-high heat, add the fritters, cook for 5 minutes on each side, arrange on a platter and serve.

Nutrition:

Calories 209;

Fat 11.2 g;

Fiber 3 g;

Carbs 4.4 g;

Protein 4.8 g

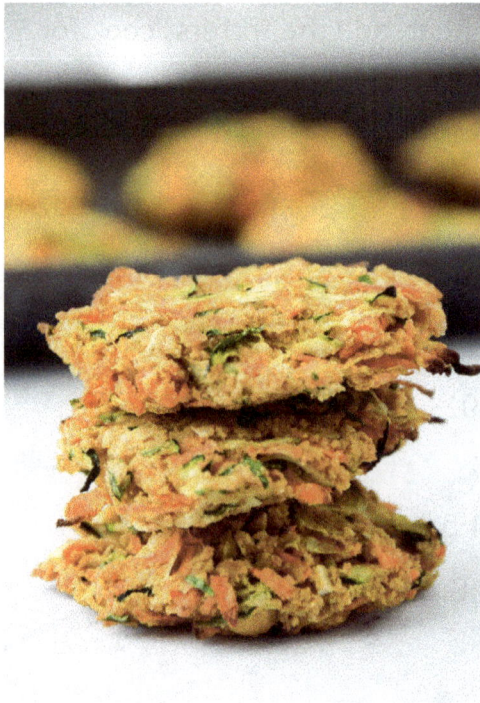

White Bean Dip

Preparation Time: 10 minutes

Cooking Time: 0 minute

Servings: 4

Ingredients:

- 15 oz. canned white beans, drained and rinsed
- 6 oz. canned artichoke hearts, drained and quartered
- 4 garlic cloves, minced
- 1 tbsp. basil, chopped
- 2 tbsp. olive oil
- Juice of ½ lemon
- Zest of ½ lemon, grated
- Salt and black pepper to the taste

Directions:

1. In your food processor, combine the beans with the artichokes and the rest of the ingredients except the oil and pulse well.
2. Add the oil gradually, pulse the mix again, divide into cups and serve as a party dip.

Nutrition:

Calories 274;

Fat 11.7 g;

Carbs 18.5 g;

Protein 16.5 g

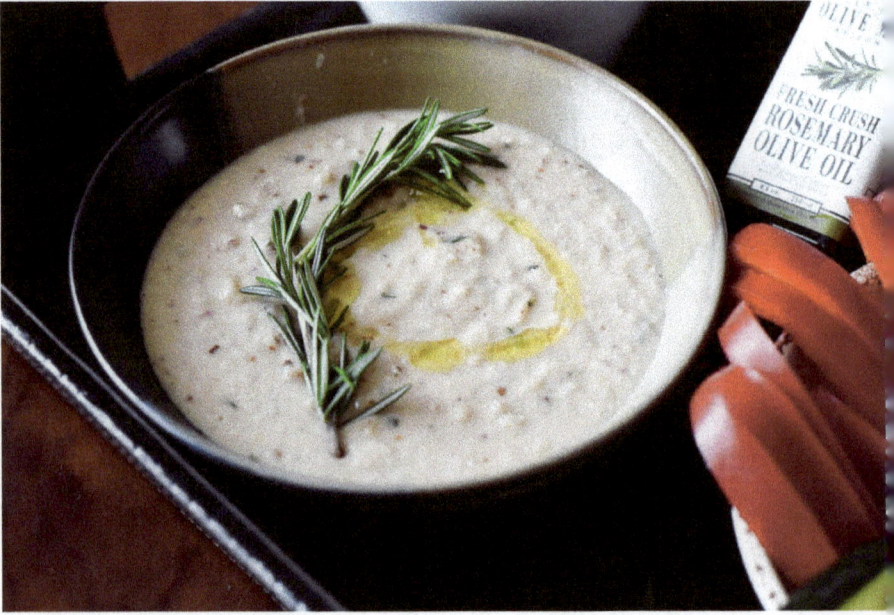

Eggplant Dip

Preparation Time: 10 minutes

Cooking Time: 40 minutes

Servings: 4

Ingredients:

- 1 eggplant, poked with a fork
- 2 tbsp. tahini paste
- 2 tbsp. lemon juice
- 2 garlic cloves, minced
- 1 tbsp. olive oil
- Salt and black pepper to the taste
- 1 tbsp. parsley, chopped

Directions:

1. Put the eggplant in a roasting pan, bake at 400° F for 40 minutes, cool down, peel and transfer to your food processor.
2. Add the rest of the ingredients except the parsley, pulse well, divide into small bowls and serve as an appetizer with the parsley sprinkled on top.

Nutrition:

Calories 121;

Fat 4.3 g;

Carbs 1.4 g;

Protein 4.3 g

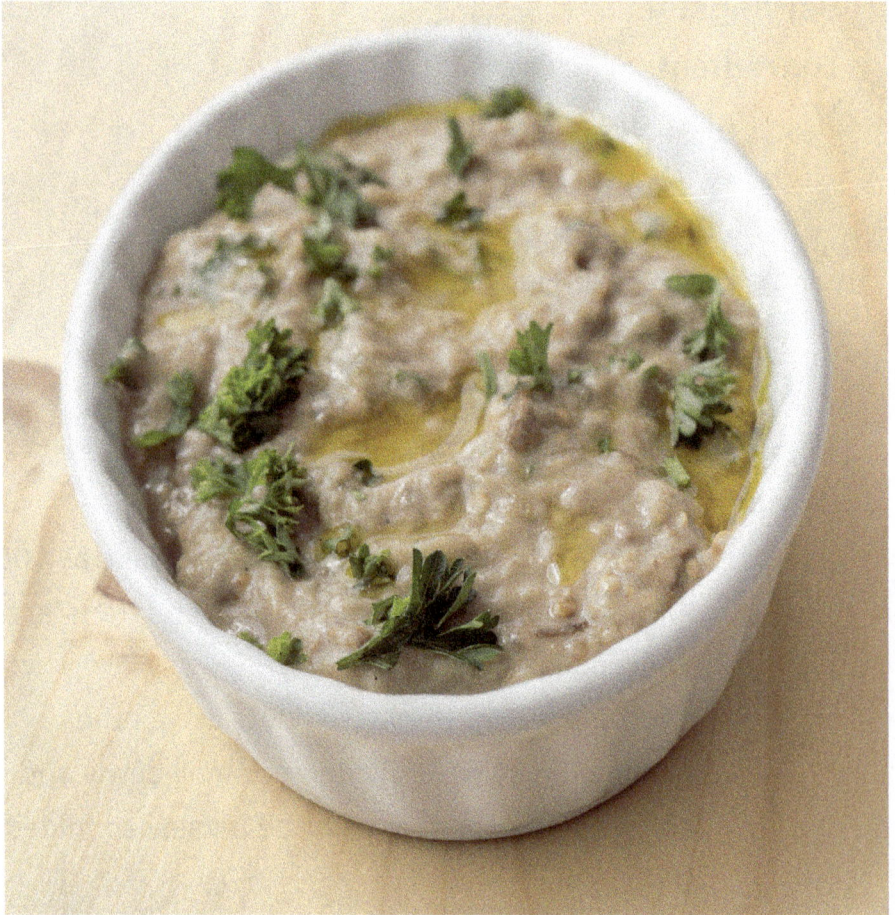

Bulgur Lamb Meatballs

Preparation Time: 10 minutes

Cooking Time: 15 minute

 Servings: 6

Ingredients:

- 1 and ½ cups Greek yogurt
- ½ tsp. cumin, ground
- 1 cup cucumber, shredded
- ½ tsp. garlic, minced
- A pinch of salt and black pepper
- 1 cup bulgur
- 2 cups water
- 1 lb. lamb, ground
- ¼ cup parsley, chopped
- ¼ cup shallots, chopped
- ½ tsp. allspice, ground
- ½ tsp. cinnamon powder
- 1 tbsp. olive oil

Directions:

1. In a bowl, combine the bulgur with the water, cover the bowl, leave aside for 10 minutes, drain and transfer to a bowl.
2. Add the meat, the yogurt and the rest of the ingredients except the oil, stir well and shape medium meatballs out of this mix.
3. Heat up a pan with the oil over medium-high heat, add the meatballs, cook them for 7 minutes on each side, arrange them all on a platter and serve as an appetizer.

Nutrition:

Calories 300;

Fat 9.6 g;

Carbs 22.6 g;

Protein 6.6 g

Cucumber Bites

Preparation Time: 10 minutes

Cooking Time: 0 minutes

Servings: 12

Ingredients:

- 1 English cucumber, sliced into 32 rounds
- 10 oz. hummus
- 16 cherry tomatoes, halved
- 1 tbsp. parsley, chopped
- 1 oz. feta cheese, crumbled

Directions:

1. Spread the hummus on each cucumber round, divide the tomato halves on each, sprinkle the cheese and parsley on to and serve as an appetizer.

Nutrition:

Calories 162;

Fat 3.4 g;

Carbs 6.4 g;

Protein 2.4 g

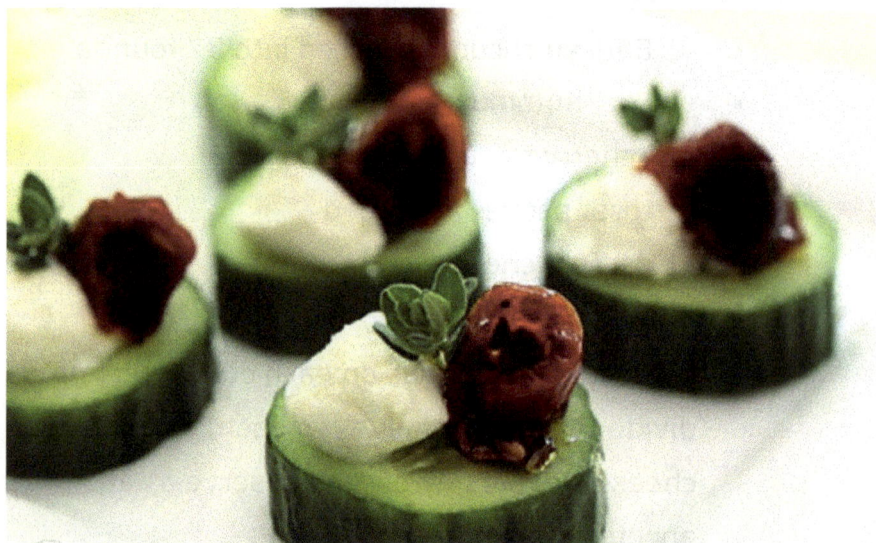

Stuffed Avocado

Preparation Time: 10 minutes

Cooking Time: 0 minute

Servings: 2

Ingredients:

- 1 avocado, halved and pitted
- 10 oz. canned tuna, drained
- 2 tbsp. sun-dried tomatoes, chopped
- 1 and ½ tbsp. basil pesto
- 2 tbsp. black olives, pitted and chopped
- Salt and black pepper to the taste
- 2 tsp. pine nuts, toasted and chopped
- 1 tbsp. basil, chopped

Directions:

2. In a bowl, combine the tuna with the sun-dried tomatoes and the rest of the ingredients except the avocado and stir.
3. Stuff the avocado halves with the tuna mix and serve as an appetizer.

Nutrition:

Calories 233;

Fat 9 g;

Carbs 11.4 g;

Protein 5.6 g

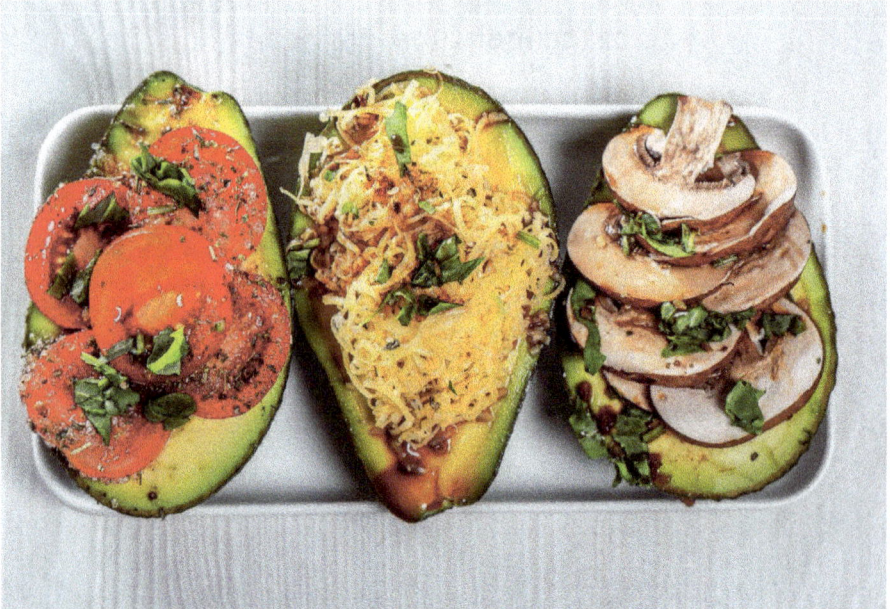

Hummus with Ground Lamb

Preparation Time: 10 minutes

Cooking Time: 15 minute

Servings: 8

Ingredients:

- 10 oz. hummus
- 12 oz. lamb meat, ground
- ½ cup pomegranate seeds
- ¼ cup parsley, chopped
- 1 tbsp. olive oil
- Pita chips for serving

Directions:

- Heat up a pan with the oil over medium-high heat, add the meat, and brown for 15 minutes stirring often.
- Spread the hummus on a platter, spread the ground lamb all over, also spread the pomegranate seeds and the parsley and serve with pita chips as a snack.

Nutrition:

Calories 133;

Fat 9.7 g;

Carbs 6.4 g;

Protein 5

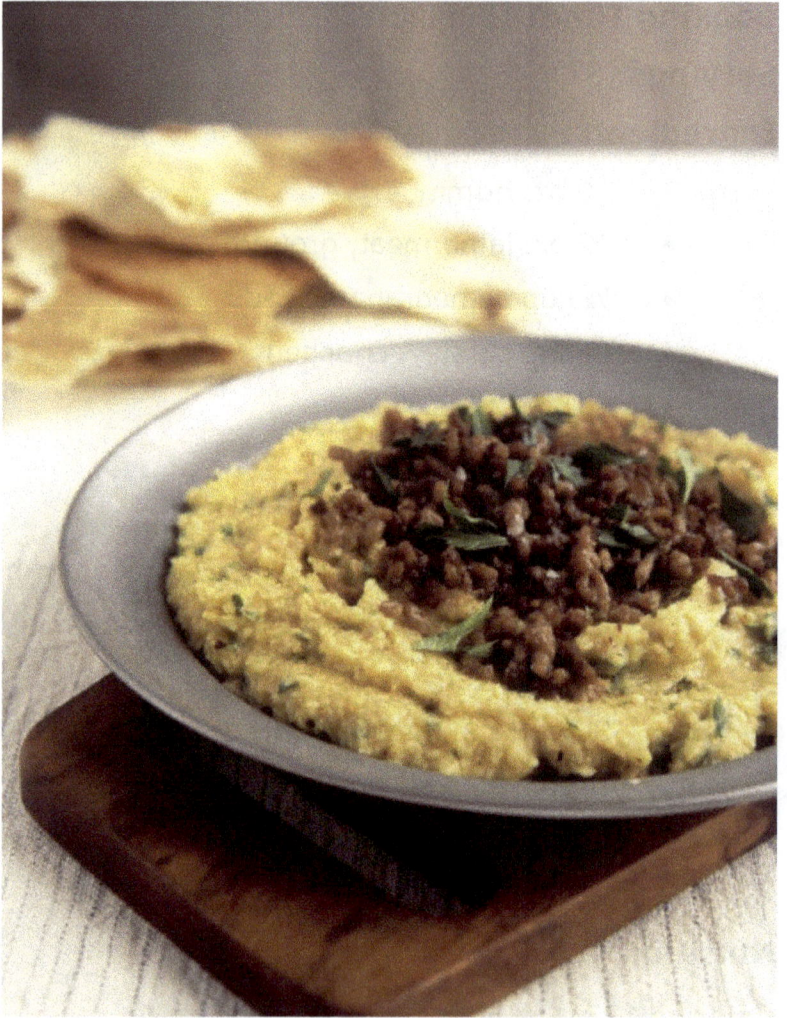

Wrapped Plums

Preparation Time: 5 minutes

Cooking Time: 0 minutes

Servings: 8

Ingredients:

1.   2 oz. prosciutto, cut into 16 pieces
2.   4 plums, quartered
3.   1 tbsp. chives, chopped
4.   A pinch of red pepper flakes, crushed

Directions:

- Wrap each plum quarter in a prosciutto slice, arrange them all on a platter, sprinkle the chives and pepper flakes all over and serve.

Nutrition:

Calories 30;

Fat 1 g;

Carbs 4 g;

Protein 2 g

Cucumber Sandwich Bites

Preparation Time: 5 minutes

Cooking Time: 0 minutes

Servings: 12

Ingredients:

1. 1 cucumber, sliced
2. 8 slices whole wheat bread
3. 2 tbsp. cream cheese, soft
4. 1 tbsp. chives, chopped
5. ¼ cup avocado, peeled, pitted and mashed
6. 1 tsp. mustard
7. Salt and black pepper to the taste

Directions:

1. Spread the mashed avocado on each bread slice, also spread the rest of the ingredients except the cucumber slices.
2. Divide the cucumber slices on the bread slices, cut each slice in thirds, arrange on a platter and serve as an appetizer.

Nutrition:

Calories 187;

Fat 12.4 g;

Carbs 4.5 g;

Protein 8.2 g

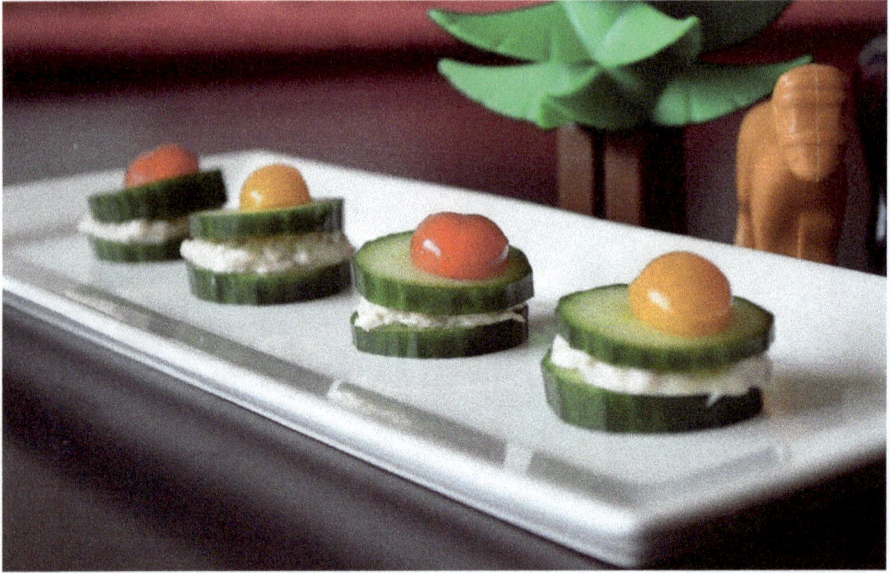